<u>New!</u>

Weightshaping

Body Sculpting and Human Performance

An Instruction Manual for Weight Training, Eating Behavior And Aerobic Exercise

by

McDaniel

Copyright 2002 by Don McDaniel and eBooksOnDisk.com

All rights reserved. No part of this book may be reproduced or transmitted in any way form or by any means, electronic or transmitted, including photo-copying, recording or by any information or retrieval system, without written permission from the publisher.

Don McDaniel
1503 Rivers Street
Pensacola, Florida 32514
Printed in the United States of America

ISBN 0-9719101-4-6

ACKNOWLEDGMENTS

Thanks to Mrs. Jan Condle, Mrs. Karen Young and Mrs. Brandy Foxworth for the exercise demonstrations and Golds Gym of Pensacola, Florida for the use of their facilities.

"The ad on the back of the comic book promised that if I sent $1.00 along with the coupon they would send the instructions on how not to be a 98-pound weakling and get sand kicked in my face. Mr. Atlas used the instructions and was pictured with muscles and girls. I sent the dollar and the coupon. I got the instructions. They forgot the muscles and the girls."

"A Disappointed Kid"

CONTENTS

PART 1

Resistance Training

Weightshaping: A Definition

Prologue

Introduction

CHAPTER	Page
1 WEIGHTSHAPING: Why?	1
2 Age and Gender	5
3 Muscles	7
Function	7
Fibers	8
Fiber Types	10
Fiber Recruitment	11
Energy Costs	12
4. Body Fat	13
5. Strength, Power and Muscle Size	15
6. Lifting	19
Lifting: One or Two	20
Form	21
7. Equipment	23
Machines	23
Work Weights	26
8. Training	29
<u>The Rule</u>	29
The Eight Variables	29
Phases	33
Safety	34

Contents (cont)

9.	Warm-Up, Stretching & Calisthenics	35
10.	The Resistance Exercises	43
11.	Training Programs and Records	63
	Basic Conditioning	65
	Performance	74
	Pre-Fatigue and Exhaust	82
	Circuit Training	84
	Body Sculpting(Body Building)	90
	Strength(Power)Training	116
	Additional Training Records	127

Part 2

Eating Behavior

12.	Correcting Eating Misbehavior	133
	Nutrients	136
	Diets	140
	Weight or Fat	142
	The How and the What	144
	Good Nutrition for Good Years	145
	Body Sculpting and Eating Behavior	145

Part 3

Aerobic Exercise

13.	Aerobic (Endurance) Exercise	147
	Heart Rate	149
	Getting Started	153
	The Timeless Exercise	154
14.	Aerobic How To	157
	Think F.I.T.	157
15.	Power and Endurance	161

WEIGHTSHAPING

A Definition

Weight:

    1. Exercise equipment which is lifted; as in weight.

Lifting:

    2. A measure of the force of gravity.

Shaping:

    1. To modify.

    2. To give a particular form to.

    3. The process of getting in shape; as in fitness.

WEIGHTSHAPING:

    An inclusive term for using weight training, aerobic exercise and correct behavior to enhance **Form, Function and Physiology**.

PROLOGUE

WEIGHTSHAPING is for the layperson and student who wants and needs information about resistance training, aerobic exercise and eating behavior.

There are many books written about these activities. Some of them are academic texts. Most of them are for the public. The academic texts tell us the why, but the how is often not clear. The texts for the public seldom tell us the why and may be inaccurate about the how. **WEIGHTSHAPING** attempts to combine and clarify the two approaches. It is one of the few instruction manuals for the layperson which turns the current scientific why into the practical how of weight training.

It is, hopefully, an easy-to-read compilation of current knowledge and its application. In many ways, it is also a recipe book. It outlines the goals, what to do, how much and when. It gives the data necessary to make intelligent decisions about what we ought to do. An understanding of how the body functions and fundamentals is essential to knowing what to do and how to do it.

There is a program for everyone and a guide for every day of each program.

There is no claim that these instructions contain a translation of all of the available scientific data. But it does come close; close without confusing the issue.

Choose your goals, pick the program, follow the recipe and keep your records. It works if you do.

1
WEIGHT TRAINING: WHY?

The question is often asked, "What is the best way to train with weights?" The answer is simple: no one knows. We are still learning. What we have learned is that some ways are better than other ways. The better way is specific to what we wish to accomplish, be it to have the body beautiful or be the world's strongest person.

Whatever the goal, it can be accomplished by training the muscles. But each goal requires that the muscles be used in a different and specific way. For this we first need an understanding of how muscles work.

Only a few years ago athletes were advised not to lift weights. No one was suggesting that youth, men over 40 or women of any age should even consider a lifting program. Until recently the majority of the medical community advocated aerobic exercise to the exclusion of any type of resistance training.

Now it is the rare athlete who is not lifting for performance. Young people are weight training. Women and men of all ages are "pumping iron."

Why the change? Is there new information? No. Contrary to current opinion, the data has been available for years. Experienced people knew and told us of the benefits of weight training long before we were receptive. But, as with most ideas, it took time and additional confirmation to convince us.

For the past two decades the majority of research and opinion has been directed toward aerobic exercise. It is interesting to note that this is in spite of the fact that most of our activities are anaerobic (without oxygen). Resistance training using weights is now advocated as outlined in WEIGHTSHAPING for the most basic of reasons: it works.

It works because it enhances:

FORM by

- Maximizing fat loss
- Improving posture
- Sculpting the body

FUNCTION through

- Increasing muscle power
- Strengthening connective tissue
- Helping to prevent musculoskeletal injury
- Enhancing anaerobic stamina
- Facilitating movement

PHYSIOLOGY to

- Elevate metabolism and calorie burn
- Prevent the loss of and increase lean body mass
- Decrease the risk of the bone thinning disease osteoporosis

The question is often asked, "What is the best way to train with weights?" The answer is simple: no one knows. We are still learning. What we have learned is that some ways are better than other ways. The better way is specific to what we wish to accomplish, be it to have the body beautiful or be the world's strongest person.

Whatever the goal, it can be accomplished by training the muscles. But each goal requires that the muscles be used in a different and specific way. For this we first need an understanding of how muscles work.

2
AGE AND GENDER

Much of the popular literature emphasizes different programs for the young and not-so-young and for men and women. While it is true that there are different levels of flexibility, strength, power and recovery time, it is also true that all bodies function the same way. The principles used for the WEIGHTSHAPING programs are applicable for all ages and both sexes.

3

MUSCLES

Function

The human body has more than 400 voluntary muscles. There are big ones, little ones, short ones and long ones. But no matter what the size, they all do the same thing in the same way. They move us. Most of the muscles move bones. These muscles are called the anti-gravity muscles. They keep the bones in what is called "the upright and mobile posture." Without the muscles, the bones would collapse with the pull of gravity. The muscles move us by having one end attached to a bone and the other end attached to another bone. (A few muscles attach to connective tissue.) The two bones are connected by a joint. A muscle contracting causes the two ends of the muscle to come closer together causing the bones to change their position by swiveling at the joint.

Muscles do not push, they only pull. It is the pulling of the bones that causes movement.

Muscles do not move in isolation. When a muscle contracts and shortens across one side of a joint, the muscle on the other side of the joint must lengthen. Movements are performed by several muscles acting together. They act together in two ways. One way is for two or more muscles to pull on the same bone. The other way is for a muscle, or muscles, to be anchors. An example is when we bend at the waist and use our arms to lift a weight. The arms may do the actual lifting, but the back and stomach muscles contract in order to anchor the upper body.

SUMMARY: 1. Muscles pull, not push.

2. Muscles do not act in isolation. They act together.

FIBERS

Each muscle consists of many fibers. Think of a muscle as having 100 fibers, although they usually have many more. It is these 100 fibers going from bone to bone which we call a muscle. To understand how these fibers act to create the force necessary to move the bones, the first thing to know is that a muscle, or more accurately the fibers, contracts all the way, or it does not contract at all. It's called the "all or nothing principle." To illustrate with what is admittedly an over-simplification, if the muscle with 100 fibers is used to lift a light weight, we may need only 10 of the 100 fibers. The 10 fibers contracting all the way produce enough strength to lift the light weight. The other 90 fibers are not used. To lift a heavier weight, we may need 50 of the one hundred fibers, leaving 50 not used. The number of fibers used depends on the weight of the object to be lifted. If a weight is lifted more than once, the number of fibers used will increase. Back to the example of lifting a weight which requires the use of only 10 fibers. To lift the weight once, we use the 10 fibers. If the lift is repeated enough times, the 10 fibers will fatigue. To continue the repetitions, another 10 of the 100 fibers are contracted. When this second set of 10 is fatigued, another 10 are used until the number of repetitions result in using maybe 60 of the 100 fibers, 10 at a time, (Once again, this is an over-simplification for illustrative purposes.) A muscle which has been trained this way, low weights and high repetitions, has difficulty lifting a heavy weight requiring 90 fibers. Using only 10 fibers at a time, the muscle is not trained to use 90 at the same time.

The amount of weight which can be lifted is dependent upon the number of fibers trained at the same time. That is not to say there is not an increase in strength as a result of using low weights and many repetitions. There is an increase in strength, but not as much as when the training is done with a heavy weight, or stated more correctly, when using a large number of fibers at the same time. If the low weight, high repetition training is not the best way to increase strength, it does have its advantages. A fiber which is "contracted," "shortened," and "exercised" repetitively does increase the size of its cross sectional diameter. As the fiber increases in size, there is an increase in strength, but the major advantage is its increased bulk. The fibers which are used to lift a light weight 20 times a day for many days may be larger than they would be if the fibers are used to lift a heavy weight only a few times once a day for the same number of days, but they probably would not be as strong. There is no clear evidence as to the exact process which leads to increasing muscle size. Increase in size is probably a function of total workload rather than a specific training program.

SUMMARY: 1. A muscle is made up of many different fibers.

2. A fiber either contracts all the way or not at all.

3. The number of fibers used together determines the amount of strength produced.

4. The number of times - repetitions - a fiber is contracted, determines its size.

5. Light weights plus many repetitions produce good increases in muscles size but less than optimal strength gains.

6. Heavy weights with a few repetitions produce superior increases in strength

Fiber Types

There are three major muscle fiber types: slow-twitch, fast-twitch and intermediate. Slow-twitch fibers do just that: they contract more slowly than the fast-twitch fibers. Also, they can contract more often before becoming fatigued. The slow-twitch fibers are more suitable for endurance activities. Fast-twitch fibers are used for power movements and are not the best for endurance. With weight training, the fast-twitch fibers will increase in size more than will the slow-twitch fibers. Intermediate fibers posses some of the properties of both the slow and fast twitch fibers.

The percentage of slow-twitch and fast-twitch fibers in a muscle is probably determined genetically. There is no reason to believe that weight training can change a slow-twitch or intermediate fiber to one possessing the qualities of the fast-twitch fiber. However, it may be that the intermediate and fast-twitch fibers can, with endurance training, take on some of the functional aspects of the slow-twitch fiber.

SUMMARY: 1. Slow-twitch fibers are for endurance activities.

2. Fast twitch fibers are for more explosive movements such as weight training.

3. The percent of fiber in each category may be determined genetically

5. Weight training probably does not increase the number of fast-twitch fibers.

Fiber Recruitment

A signal goes from the nerve cell to the muscle fibers. The fibers contract after receiving the nerve signal. One nerve cell, through its many branches, may activate many muscle fibers. This combination of a nerve cell and its branches, plus the fibers it activates, is called a motor unit. A muscle has many motor units. The activation of the motor units is called recruitment. The number of motor units recruited is dependent upon the weight to be lifted. When the motor unit is recruited, the fibers follow the "all or nothing" principle of contraction. Lifting a light weight requires relatively few units recruited. Lifting a heavy weight requires the recruitment of more units. The number of motor units recruited and the frequency of their activation determines amount of force produced.

Much is said of attaining the proper mental concentration. Mental concentration can be defined as the correct anticipation of the amount of effort needed to lift a particular weight. The anticipation results in the recruiting of the number of motor units necessary to produce the required force. The more fibers recruited and the more rapid their contraction the greater is the strength. Much of this is the result of having the ability to "concentrate." Also, muscles are activated by sensors which relay information on the amount of force needed.

Apparently, training can increase the ability to recruit more fibers and increase the frequency of their stimulation. An example of this is when a person begins weight training. The muscles show very little, if any, increase in size after the first few weeks but may exhibit significant strength gains. The increase is probably the result of recruiting more fibers.

SUMMARY: 1. The nerve and the muscle fibers it serves are

2. Activation of the motor unit is called recruitment.

3. The number of motor units recruited determines the weight which can be lifted.

4. Mental concentration along with sensory feedback is the basis of recruitment.

5. Fiber recruitment is the basis of strength.

6. Training may enhance recruitment.

ENERGY COSTS

Large muscles such as the thigh, buttocks and back can not only lift more than the small ones, but they also burn more calories and are more fatigue resistant. The number of calories burned is dependent upon the size of the muscle being exercised. Large muscles use more calories than small ones. For example, squats which exercise the large leg muscles are more calorie costly than arm curls which use the small biceps muscle. Beginning a weight lifting workout by using the small muscles may have them too fatigued to adequately hold the weights for the large muscle exercises. In most workouts it is more productive to work the large muscles first followed by exercises for the small muscles.

SUMMARY: 1. Large muscles can work longer with greater strength than small muscles.

2. <u>Fatigue the large muscles first and then the small ones</u>.

3. Large muscles burn more calories than small ones.

4

BODY FAT

One of the most sought after results of any exercise program is to lose body fat. While the stated goal may be health, function or to feel good, in fact, looking good is a prime consideration. For most of us this means having that lean "well defined" appearance. A prevalent notion is that if the muscles get larger through training they will be well defined, but this is not necessarily true. If a person has very little body fat to begin with then definition is probable, especially for males. Most females, because of relatively small amounts of the hormone testosterone, will not significantly increase muscle size. For both sexes larger muscles will not be defined if they are hidden by excess fat.

Fat control is essential for exhibiting the musculature!

Exercise elevates our calorie expenditure and, therefore, burns more fat than when we are sedentary. Aerobic exercise burns more calories during exercise than does anaerobic exercise. But, apparently, anaerobic exercise such as resistance training causes the body to burn more calories during non-exercise time than does aerobic exercise. Remember, muscles account for a significant number of the calories we burn and are called the calorie burning machines of the body. Resistance training increases not only muscle size but probably metabolic rate resulting in more muscle activity and, therefore, more calories used. Most data indicate that energy costs are significantly raised as a result of resistance training. But, and this is an important point to understand, it is difficult to control fat levels over the long-term by exercise alone. An example: The so-called average person burns about 100 calories walking one mile. One pound of fat is 3500 calories. That means one must walk 35 miles to lose one pound of fat! That is a lot of exercise. To control fat levels one must control eating behavior in addition to exercising. For effective fat loss, appropriate exercise and good eating behavior, not misbehavior, are essential.

It is not the purpose of these instructions to cover diet and eating behavior. To learn more on the subject you may wish to consult with a registered dietician. Also, BODY FAT: A LOSER'S MANUAL by this author covers the subject in depth.

5

STRENGTH, POWER AND MUSCLE SIZE

There is a great deal of misunderstanding about the difference between strength and power. There may be even more confusion about how these two relate to increasing muscle size, i.e., the goal of the serious body builder, and the methods necessary to train for each. Unfortunately, understanding the concepts and their appropriate applications is rarely, very rarely, found within the "fitness" community. This discussion may entail more than you wish to know, somewhat like asking what time it is and the person tells you how to build a clock! But there are two very good reasons why this is important for each of us to know. First, it enables us to understand how to construct our own resistance training program, and second, it will allow you to know whether or not the "fitness expert" has the slightest idea about what they are trying to impress you with!

Strength is the ability to move force through a distance ($S = F \times D$). Think of force as resistance. That force may be in the form of a barbell, dumbbell or body weight. The greater the weight (weight is a measure of force, ; e.g., the force of gravity) the greater the force. (As an aside, force is the product of mass times acceleration ($F = M \times A$) with mass being the ability to overcome inertia, that is, no movement.) Note that the time it takes to move the force a distance is not in the equation. To be successful, most human movements require a time frame. Try taking three hours to lift a very heavy object overhead! How well could you run if each forward step took two minutes? Extremes examples, but they make the point.

Take the strength equation and divide it by time. This makes it power. For simplification, do the division. If we wish to find the velocity (speed) of any movement, divide the distance by how long it takes to make the trip. Do this to the power equation and power becomes the result of multiplying force by the velocity, ($P = F \times V$).

This makes power the application of strength! It also, and this is important, means that all human movement is power! Do not all of our movements involve moving a force with a certain velocity? Of course. So it is not a question of whether a movement is strength or power, but a matter of how much power. Another way of stating the obvious is that we do not train to create power but to increase it.

When someone says they wish to get stronger they are in reality saying they wish to get more powerful.

How do we get this increase in power? We must revisit the equation $P = F \times V$. Obviously, if we increase force and keep the velocity the same, the power goes up, and doing the opposite, keeping the force the same and increasing the velocity also yields more power. Of course increasing both force and velocity does the same. These three ways of upping our power output are valid only to a point. Think about it. If the force increases too much (e.g., the weight is too heavy) the velocity goes down and the power may not increase, increase only slightly, or even decrease. To significantly increase the velocity it is necessary that the force be diminished.

Consider this example; If a runner gets to large the speed suffers. (Remember the force equation; the mass is too large to increase acceleration and the force goes down.) For the speed to go up the weight must not become excessive.

Most data indicate that producing a force (moving a weight) about 40 - 45 % of the maximum force of which you are capable of doing for one repetition is the best force amount to be moved at the highest possible velocity and, therefore, produces the most power.

The training programs for strength, power and increasing muscle size are straightforward.

High volume, which means the weight can be lifted for many repetitions and sets, emphasizes strength and increasing muscle size. Low volume, weight lifted relatively few reps and sets, emphasizes increasing power. It is not a question of either or, but one of emphasis.

Increasing muscle size, body building, is a function of sustained contraction (stimulation), hence high volume, reps and sets, with low velocity (done slowly). Body builders will often swear that they got big muscles by lifting heavy weights. Not so! Big muscles are the product of sustained contraction, regardless of the weight.

This information on strength, power and increasing muscle size is the basis for program design in this instruction manual.

6

LIFTING

CONTRACTION AND ACTION

The how of lifting is as important as the how much. How a lift is performed, slow or fast, depends on what the lifter wishes to accomplish.

There is some evidence which suggests that for Body Sculpting, lifts done slowly - sustained stimulation - with proper form may be more beneficial than lifts done rapidly. The opposite may be true for Power and Performance Training.

Four different speed combinations (methods) for the lifting (concentric) and the lowering (eccentric) of the weight can be considered. Isometric action is when the fibers produce force but do not change the joint angle. It should be used at the conclusion of the concentric lift.

1. Slow concentric (three-second minimum) and slow eccentric (three-second minimum) are recommended for Body Sculpting and can be a part of Power Training.

2. Moderate concentric and slow eccentric (two-second minimum) are recommended for Basic Conditioning and Power Training and can be a part of Circuit Training and Body Sculpting.

3. Fast speeds for concentric and moderate for eccentric are used primarily for performance and power training.

4. For body sculpting, at the conclusion of each concentric lift hold an isometric action for a full second.

Lifts should be done using a full range of motion. In Body Sculpting, it is often recommended that the lift not be done to full motion in order to maintain constant tension. There is some merit to this, but it will have a tendency to shorten the muscles and is not recommended for the other training programs.

Important: For performance training the best results may be obtained by doing the concentric lift with maximum speed, regardless of the weight used. For developing complex motor skills necessary for sports it may be more beneficial to do both light weights with high repetitions and heavy weights with low repetitions at maximum speed with the motion duplicating as closely as possible the desired sport movements.

Lifting: One or Two?

One of the most neglected aspects of lifting is the alternating use of the arms and legs. Traditionally, almost all lifting instructions illustrate the use of both arms or both legs moving in the same motion at the same time.

How many movements require both arms or both legs to move in the same direction at the same time? Very few. When an arm or leg moves in one direction, the other arm or leg moves in another, usually the opposite direction. that is the way we are wired to function. So why train with the limbs going in the same direction? If strength (power) is demonstrated by a two-arm or two-leg movement such as competitive weight lifting, then, obviously, we should train that way. But if the goal is to demonstrate power and performance, why not train our bodies in the way they are designed to function?

Remember, training is specific. Training the limbs to go in the same direction is training them for a movement that is usually not specific to the way we function.

When appropriate, the illustrations for lifts will be given for using the limbs moving in the same direction at the same time and alternating the movements.

Alternating movements are recommended for performance training and may be used for other programs.

FORM

"Use good form" is one of the most misunderstood concepts in resistance training. More often than not those who advise you to use good form are not aware of what it means or why.

Good form is specific to one's goals. Proper form for a body builder should be for maintaining constant tension, which facilitates muscle stimulation for increasing size. This means not using ballistic motion, i.e. using a swinging move or utilizing speed to accomplish a lift, because tension is reduced.

Remember training is specific. Try training specifically for performance without using a ballistic motion. Furthermore, try thinking of an athletic or performance move that does not require a ballistic move. Weight lifting moves such as the clean and jerk and snatch require good anatomical form for balance, the production of power and getting the most out of speed movements. These are ballistic moves!

There is a great deal made of using proper form for injury prevention. What may be of equal or greater significance is building the muscle structure to compensate for deviations from the so-called proper form. If there is a structural weakness, the use of support devices such as weight belts and braces are questionable. It usually makes more sense to develop the muscles in the affected area. You may wish to consider that the majority of people who use weight belts do so for reasons other than support. Most of the time they are for making the midsection look smaller or because they think it looks "professional." Most non-rigid leg and arm braces have very little to do with anatomical integrity; they are strictly for looks!

Many effective lifting movements are judged to violate the accepted tenants of good form when, in fact, the form used is necessary for accomplishing the lift as well as being the most beneficial for training. To develop power for performance in a wide variety of sport and work tasks one must consider the basic rule of resistance training; move many different fibers in many different planes of motion. An example: I was working out in a hospital wellness center prior to making a two-hour presentation to the membership and was lifting on a seated row machine with, what for me, was a heavy weight. I used legs, arms, back and every other muscle I could recruit; obeying the resistance training principle. If I had to duplicate that movement in a real-life situation, training in that manner is the sensible way to do it. It would lessen the possibility of injury as well as facilitate the ability to perform. Two very fine exercise directors at the center were observing and genuinely horrified. To them, everything was done wrong. I spent a good deal of time explaining, or trying to. It did no good. They had read the equipment manufacturers instructions on good form and to them that was the gospel. What happened was that they never considered that what constitutes good form is always specific to the goal or task!

7

EQUIPMENT

Is there an ideal piece of equipment? Yes! It is called the human body. That is the piece of equipment which you must move in order to get "in shape." As for other types of equipment, you should move the equipment, not have the equipment move you. Once it is understood that no piece of equipment, other than the body, does anything for you, that it is what you do with the equipment that matters, only then can any equipment be put to good use. When considering which equipment to use in addition to the body, an understanding is needed of the pros and cons of each type.

Machines

"It is certain that there are world class athletes, body builders, and weight lifters who are the way they are as a result of using machines. It is just that we have never known one, seen one, heard of one or read of one in the reputable literature." Someone once asked about the difference between free weights (work weights) and machines. The reply was, "nothing but misinformation and the workload."

The resistance training machines discussed here should not be confused with aerobic machines, stationary apparatus and certain pulley devices.

Use a machine which is designated military or shoulder press. Set the weight load at 100 pounds. Lift it. Then lift a 100 pound barbell. The barbell will be much more difficult to lift than the same weight load on the machine. Why?

You are probably seated when using the machine and, therefore, are not using the legs and lower body to support the weight. By not using the lower body, the amount of work is reduced. Also, on a machine, the weight is in place and does not have to be lifted to a starting position. Once again there is a reduced work load. The weight in the machine is stabilized, directed and balanced. This work is done by the machine, not the body. A lift with a machine is in a groove. It is directed in one plane of motion. This limits the recruiting of fibers and, consequently, the results. Human movement will rarely be done in one plane of motion and it is even more rare to perform with a motion which corresponds to that of a machine.

Performance training can be severely limited by the use of machines. Performance training involves the use of multi-joint exercises which can not be duplicated on a machine.

Also, for high intensity contractions at the beginning of a performance there is a need for preloading. Muscles do not respond instantaneously to maximum demands. Their is a brief period needed for the processes which produce high intensity movement to become activated. This usually is in the form of an isometric action, or preload. For reasons which are beyond the scope of these instructions, most machines do not provide a preload because they are holding or supporting the weight.

For best <u>performance</u> and <u>power</u> results and greater workload (caloric burn), the muscle should not be isolated. Most machine weight training devices tend to use fewer muscles per exercise and attempt to work a muscle in isolation. For some body sculpting exercises, isolating the muscles may be of benefit.

Training is specific. If one trains on machines, one becomes more capable of training on machines. Relative to other kinds of training there is limited carry over from performance on machines to human performance.

However, using machines for certain exercises may(?) be advantageous because the movements are difficult to duplicate with work weights.

Machines can be supplemental to work weights (maybe), but cannot functionally replace them. General criteria for determining the relative usefulness of resistance training machines are:

1. If the apparatus has moving parts, the workload is reduced and a better workload can be produced with work weights.

2. If the apparatus has no moving parts, i.e., and you have to move your body weight through the exercise, such as dips and pull ups, the workload is appropriately high.

Also, the novelty of machines can be interesting and provide motivation for the beginner. For some, this advantage can outweigh the sacrifice in training results.

For people with certain types of injuries, machines may be the only viable alternative.

All of this is not to say that machines cannot produce benefits. They can. It depends on one's goals and initial condition. For the novice, anything which is more than what one has done will yield results. But for equal time invested, the results are limited when machines are compared to work weights.

Specifically, machines are not the best way to train for power or performance. Their use is better justified for certain aspects of body sculpting. (Maybe?)

Summary:
1. Resistance is stabilized and balanced by machines.
2. Motion is in a restricted plane.
3. The weight does not have to be positioned.
4. Muscles are not used in synergy.
5. Few machines provide a preload.
5. There is a relatively low workload.
6. There is limited carryover to human

Work Weights

One of the "ugliest" and least glamorous pieces of resistance training equipment, particularly for upper body exercises, is probably the most effective: the dumbbell. A close second for many upper body programs and the most effective for large muscle exercises is the barbell. Nothing else comes even close. They should be termed "work weights" rather than free weights because using them results in more work, and a higher workload yields greater results.

Remember the example that compared a 100-pound lift on the machine to the same weight lifted on the barbell? The barbell must be lifted into position supported by the muscles of the lower body, stabilized, balanced, directed, and can be varied as to plane of motion. That is a great deal more work than is required by other resistance training modalities. Carry the example one step further and do a 100-pound lift with two 50-pound dumbbells. As the barbell was more difficult than the machine, the dumbbells are a great deal more difficult than the barbell. One of the reasons for this is that there is no dominant side help with the dumbbell, plus the body is forced to stabilize, direct and balance separate weights rather than just one.

Advocates of machine training almost always defend their use with the rationale that work weights are dangerous and cause injury. Reliable data on the subject has not been made evident. After more years than should be remembered spent in gyms and weight rooms, the author suggests that the incidence of injury with work weights is no greater than any other type apparatus. Another consideration is that, for those trained on machines, the injury rate during later performance may exceed that of those trained on work weights. It could be the result of the work weight training being more specific to the task, using more planes of motion, developing the supportive muscles, training more muscle groups at the same time and producing a greater work load.

Work weights are inexpensive, almost maintenance free, and they outlast the user. Consider that many of the commercial machines that work only one body part may cost over $3000.00, but a $50.00 department store work weight will work more body parts and may be far more productive.

SUMMARY: 1. Dumbbells and Barbells (work weights) yield higher workloads than do machines.

2. Work weights train the muscles to work in unison.

3. Work weights are less costly and last longer.

8

TRAINING

THE RULE OF RESISTANCE TRAINING

Move many different muscle fibers through varying planes of motion against increasing resistance to reach an appropriate end point.

This rule is applicable to all resistance training programs. The variance is in the application and the application is specific to the goal.

There are at least eight variables in structuring a resistance program. Learn and apply these and you will join the ranks of the relatively few who are informed, and you will be capable of structuring programs for any goal or situation.

THE EIGHT VARIABLES

<u>Goal Options</u>: Body Sculpting

        Weight Lifting

        Power Lifting

        Performance Training

<u>Body Sculpting</u> has two and only two goals which are achieved by altering one's geometric configuration. The first is to enable the devotee to enjoy looking in mirrors and the second is to enjoy getting others to look at you. Functionality, power production or performance has no place in Body Sculpting.

Weight Lifting is a sport. It usually consists of clean and jerk and snatch and incorporates both force and velocity.

Power Lifting is a misnomer. The emphasis is on force - weight - and not on velocity which effectively reduces power (P=FxV) The lifts are squat, dead lift and bench press.

Performance Training can be for anything from daily living requirements to athletic performance. The goal is to increase power for any desired movement.

End Point Defined as the amount of stimulation attained for the last repetition of each set. The cell responds to stimulation not numbers. The cell must be stimulated in order to have something to adapt to. It does no good to do a number of reps if there is not adequate stimulation. This makes the question how much weight should I use moot. Use the amount of weight necessary to achieve the end point. We use three end points. Moderate which is a little more fatigue than that to which we are accustomed and is usually for beginners, elicit fatigue which is not total muscle failure but does result in a difficult last rep and is the most commonly used point and muscle failure which is used sparingly and for the reasonably well conditioned.

Lift Speed Can be concentric(contraction) or eccentric(action) or as is colloquially known, up or down, done with moderate, slow or fast speed. As a general rule all body sculpting moves are done slowly in order to sustain stimulation for increasing muscle size. In power lifting speed is irrelevant. Just do it. Weight Lifting and Performance Training range from fast up (concentric) and slow down(eccentric) to all fast moves.

Number of Repetitions The number of successive exercise movements without interruption. Many are recommended for body sculpting to increase the stimulation time and relatively few for the other programs which seek to increase motor unit recruitment(force production) .The more force required, the more motor units need to be recruited which means heavier weights and therefore fewer reps. How many are many and few? Contrary to popularly held opinion, and it=s just that - opinion - no one knows! There are too many variables to even come close to being specific. The number recommended in this instruction manual are simply best guesses. Many may be 10-15 and few may be anything less. It is fairly certain that a very large number of reps, maybe more than 20, results in a shift toward aerobic metabolism(endurance) and away from anaerobic metabolism(short term, high force).

Number of Sets. A set is doing the same exercise for a given number of reps. As is true for repetitions the number of sets is rather arbitrary. As a general rule body sculpting requires a greater number sets than does performance training or for the sport of weight lifting, although this is not a hard and fast rule. Obviously, the more reps and sets requires lighter weights. Heavier weights result in fewer sets and reps.

Time Between Sets An adequate fuel supply is necessary to create the high force and velocity exercises necessary for performance and sport training. Replenishment of these fuels can take from two to five minutes. Conversely, body sculpting is not concerned with force and velocity and so fuel stores are a minor consideration.

Thirty to 90 seconds may be sufficient for body building.

Frequency If only we knew! Frequency is dependent upon the work load of the previous workout. It is a mistake to do too much too soon so that the body does not have time to recuperate. Remember, cells must have time to adapt to the stimulus of exercise. Without adaptation there is no progress. Maximum stimulation may require only two workouts a week. Very low stimulation can sometimes allow for six workouts a week. The key is listen to the body. If sleep patterns are disrupted, there is excessive urination, abnormal mood swings, elevated heart rate and most importantly a general feeling of malaise and fatigue then the body is saying let me rest! One need not have all of these symptoms to be warned. Often times one is a strong enough signal. Young obsessives tend to listen to peer groups and not biology. So, how frequently is just right? When you feel like it!

Duration Any one exercise program can become boring and tiresome if it=s duration is too long. For the average exerciser six weeks may be the maximum and quite possibly much shorter than that.

PHASES

One of the more progressive training programs is called phases or cycles. Designed to provide a variety of stimuli from high volume to high intensity, phases can be for periods ranging from weeks to years. An example of a phase program for the recreational exerciser could be something like this:

Goal: Performance Training

	Volume	AR	Intensity	AR	Peak	AR	Performance
End Point	Mod.		EF		EF/MF		MF
Lift Speed	Mod.		FastC.ModE		FastC.SlowE.		Fast
Reps	10-12		7-9		5-6		3-5
Sets	5-7		4-5		3-4		2-3
Time/Sets	2 Min.		2-Min		3-4 Min		3-4 Min
Frequency	4-5/Wk	3/D	EOD	3D	3-4/Wk	3D	3/Wk
Duration	5-6Wks		3-4Wks		3Wks		2Wks

*Legend: AR=active rest, Mod.=moderate, EF=elicit fatigue, MF=muscle failure, C=concentric, E=eccentric, EOD=every other day.

This basic idea can be adapted for almost any type exercise program: high volume to high intensity.

SAFETY

For any physical activity, it is prudent to follow sensible safety precautions. Although the incidence of exercise induced injury is relatively limited, the following recommendations should be adhered to.

1. If there is a history of medical problems, get a physician's clearance before beginning an exercise program.

2. Warm up and stretch before exercising. Cool down by repeating the stretching exercises.

3. Do one or two warm-up sets with reduced weight before beginning your regular program.

4. Use relatively light weights when starting a new exercise. (moderate end point)

5. Exercise through the full range of motion.

6. Do not ignore pain in or around the joints.

7. Never attempt to lift maximum loads without proper periods of training.

8. Before beginning an exercise program receive professional instructions.

9. When engaged in resistance training have one or two people as spotters.

10. Make certain that weight collars are on and secure.

11. Do not exercise when ill or injured and cease exercise at the first sign of pain.

9
Warm Up, Stretching & Calisthenics

The exercises progress from warm up to stretching to using the body's weight as resistance emphasizing movement in many planes of motion, increasing flexibility, speed and strength. Proceed at your own pace.

Reach

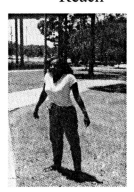

Arm Swings
All planes of motion- 5 each

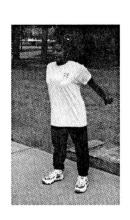
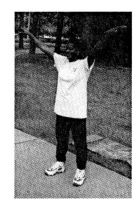

Trunk Rotation

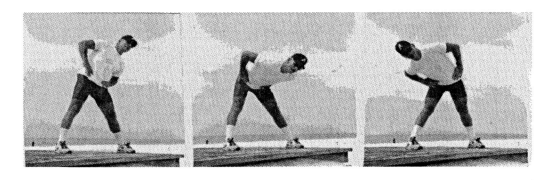

Knee Ups 5-- Each Leg

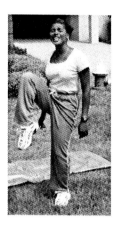

Side Squat   5 Each Leg

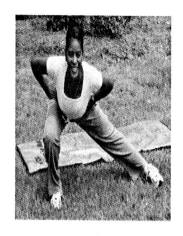

Heel Stretch   20 Seconds

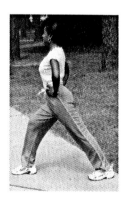

Hamstring   20 Seconds

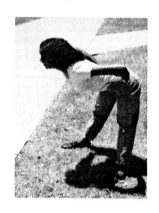

Hang Ten   20 Seconds

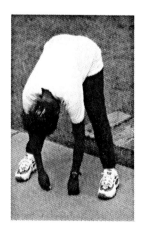

Windmill   5 Each Way

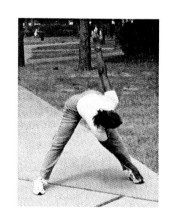

Half Squat   8

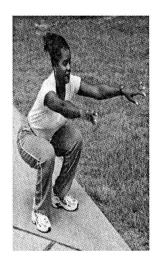

Toe Raises   8

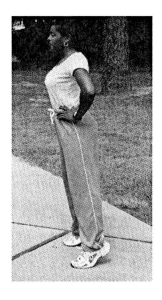

Leg Curls   5 Each

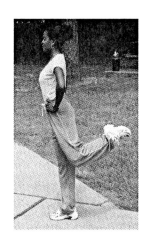

Leg Extensions 5 Each

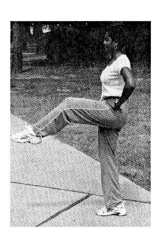

High Leg Kick   5 Each Leg

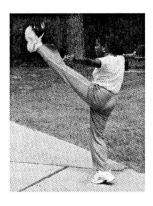

Side Straddle Hop 10 Side, 10 Front

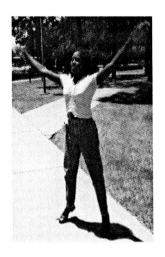

Up/Downs 5–10

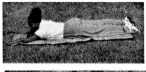
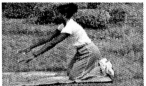
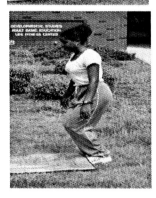

Curl Ups   10

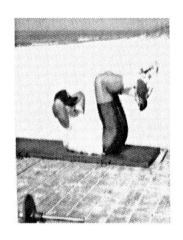
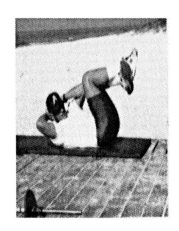
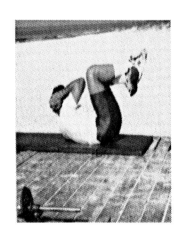

Seated Toe Touches 30 Seconds

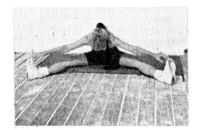

Bike Knee Ups   10 Each Leg

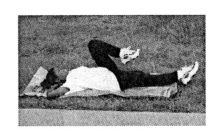

Back Extension   15 Seconds

Squat Jumps   5-10

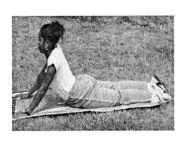
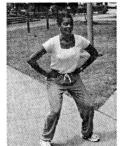
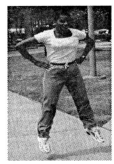
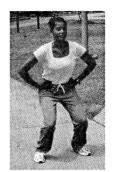

Push Ups   8-20

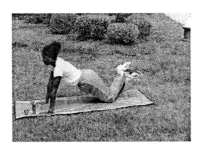
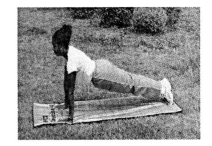

Donkey Kick   5 Each Leg

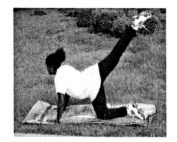

Lunge   5 Each Leg

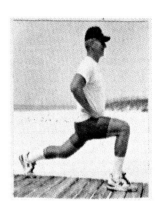

Crab Walk   4-Directional

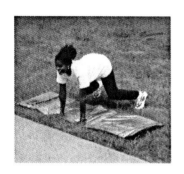
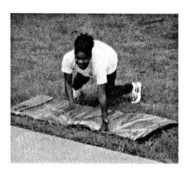

Leg Pull   30 Seconds

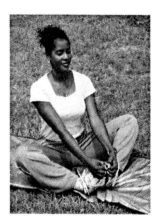

Shuffle   Two Minutes

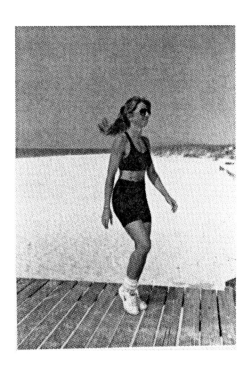

10
THE RESISTANCE EXERCISES

NOTE: This is not an all-inclusive list. You may wish to use additional supplemental exercises.

MULTIJOINT/MAJOR MUSCLE EXERCISES
Back Squats

Bar across upper back, not on the neck. Bend the knees until thighs are parallel to the floor. Keep head up and back straight. Bar kept in a vertical path.
(Top of thigh, buttocks, lower back, back of thigh, back of lower leg)

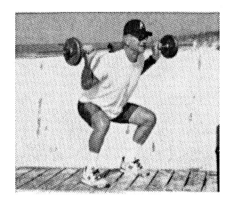

Front

Wide hand grip and high elbows. Head up and back straight. Keep bar on - vertical path.
(Lower top of thigh, buttocks, back of thigh, back of lower leg. Tends to minimize back stress.)

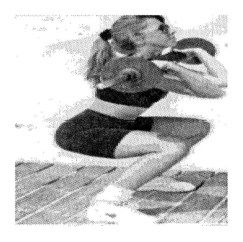

43

Lunge Squat
Same starting position as back squat. Extend up and step. Front leg vertical and thigh parallel.
(Top of thigh, buttocks, shoulders, back)

Overhead Squat
Weight overhead, do same as back squat with hands wide and arms back.

(Top of thigh, buttocks, shoulders, back)

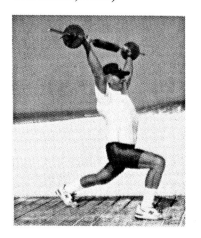 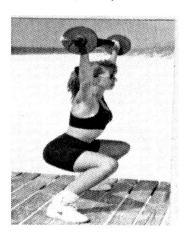

Clean Pull
Back straight, head up, shoulders ahead of bar. Heels on floor. Lift with legs. As bar clears knees lift with back and arms. Keep the bar close to the body. When the bar clears the chest the knees bend the knees lowering the body under the bar. Stand with bar resting on hands and the elbows high.
(Top of thigh, back of thigh, buttocks, back, shoulders, arms)

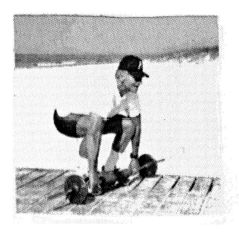 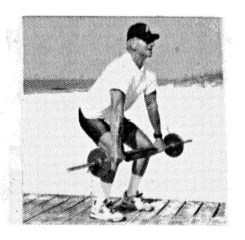

CLEAN (con't)

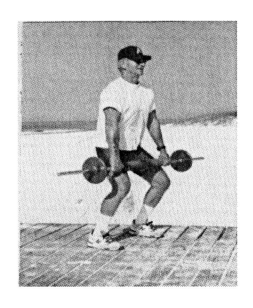
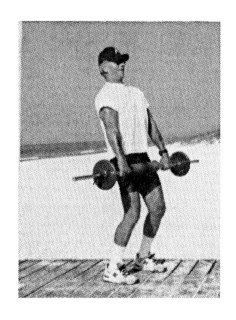
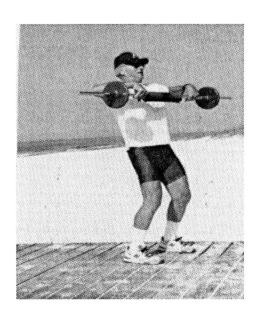
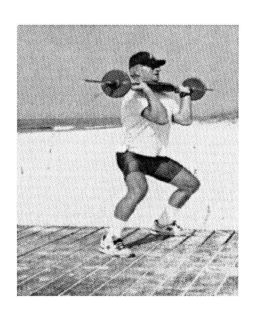

Jerk

After the clean drive upward from bent knees and extend arms. Move under the weight with a push, side split or front split. Keep the head up and looking forward.

(Top of Thigh, Shoulders, Back, Back of Upper Arm)
Push Jerk

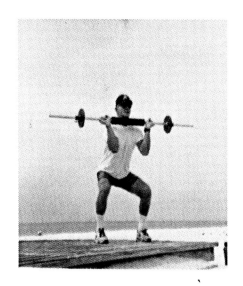
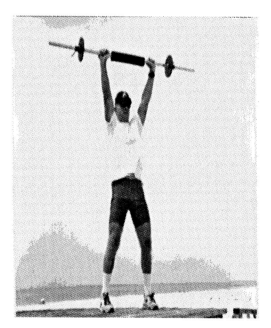

Side Split Jerk

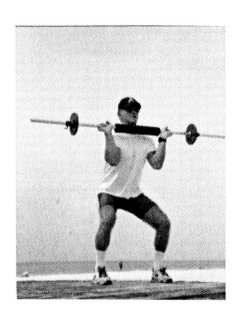
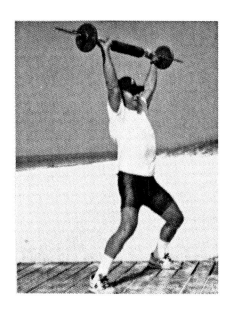

Front Split Jerk

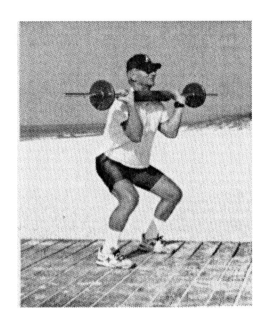 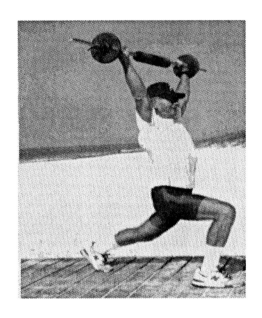

Snatch

Wide grip. Start in the same position as the Clean. Keep the arms high at the end of the pull. Keep the bar close to the body from the knees up. As the bar clears the shoulders drop under the bar with a knee bend. When the bar is overhead stand with back straight and the head forward. (Top of thigh, buttocks, back of thigh, shoulders, back, arms)

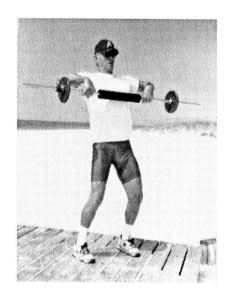
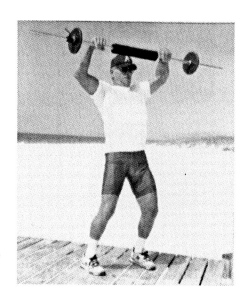
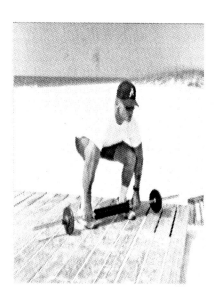
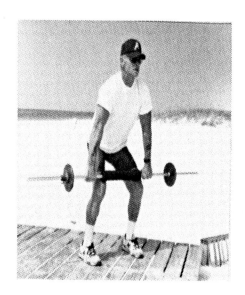

Snatch, (cont')

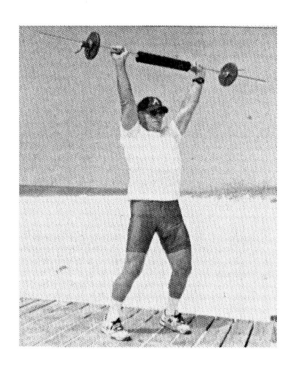

Toe Raises
Bar in same position as in squats.
Up on toes to full extension. Hold one count.

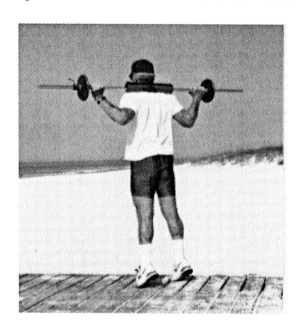

Leg Curls
Two legs or alternate legs. Heels firmly under bar.   Flex heels close to buttocks. Lower slowly.

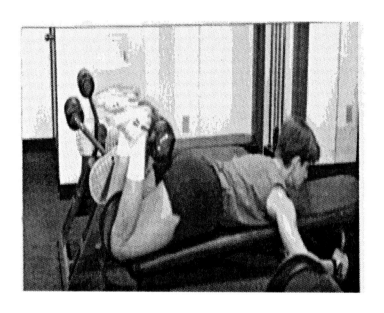

Leg Extensions
Two legs or alternate legs.
Sit upright. Extend Legs (leg) fully. Hold one count.

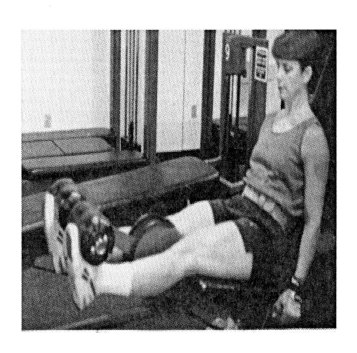

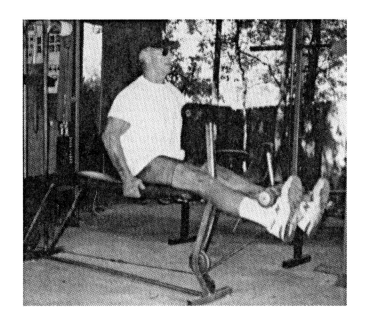

ABDOMEN

NOTE: Concentrate on intensity rather than duration. Ten to 15 repetitions are adequate. A barbell plate or a dumbbell held on the chest or behind the neck supplies the intensity for crunches. A dumbbell between the feet can be used for the basket hangs.
These devices should be added only after adapting to doing the exercises without resistance.

Crunch Sit Ups(Crunches)

(Top of stomach)

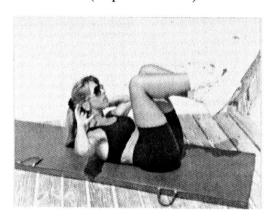

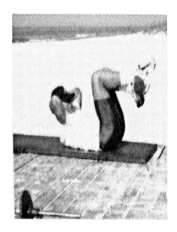 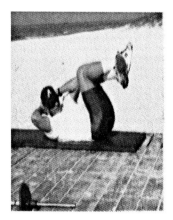 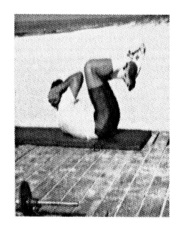

Basket Hang

Hang without swinging. Lift Knees to chest. Side hangs are done by alternating lifting knees to the elbows.
(Lower Abdomen)

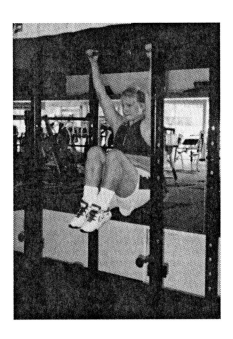
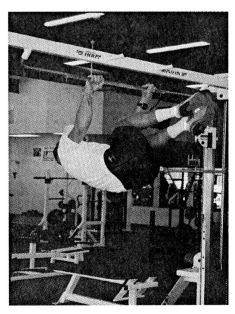

SHOULDERS

Seated Overhead Press

For body sculpting as opposed to performance training. Back, neck and head straight.

(Shoulders and back of neck)

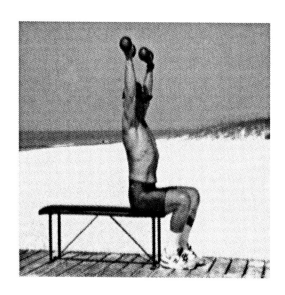

Standing Overhead Press

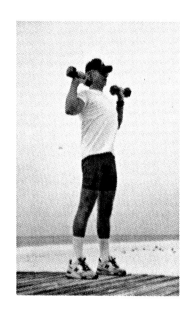
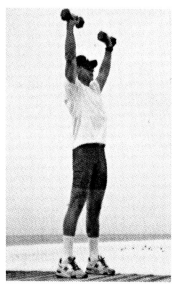
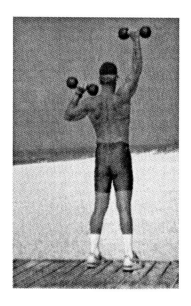

Pull Lift

Back straight. Lift weight to top of head. Use cobra grip with high elbows.
(Shoulder, side of neck and arms)

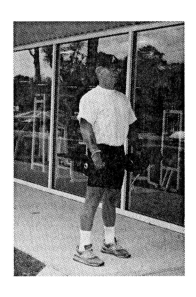 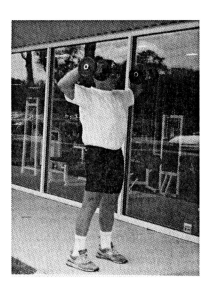

Lateral Lift

Slight bend in elbows. Lift to 45 degrees above horizontal.
(Shoulder and upper back)

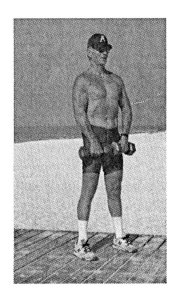 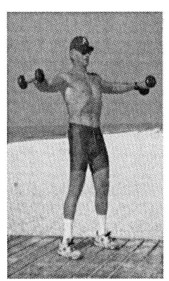 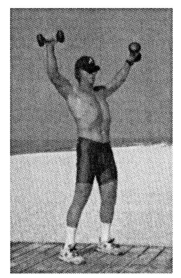

Shrugs
Two or alternate arms.
Arms straight, shoulders high.
(Top of shoulder and back of neck)

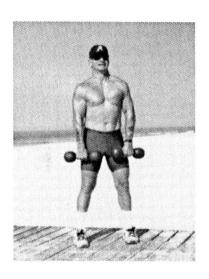 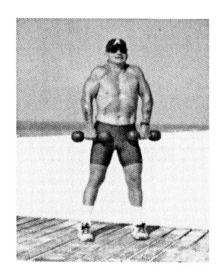

Back
Bent Row
Two or alternate arms
Knees bent. Back straight. Lift arms until elbows are above back.
(Middle and side of back)

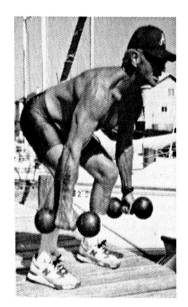 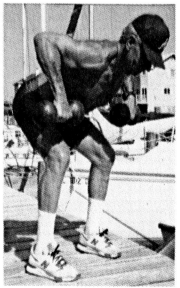 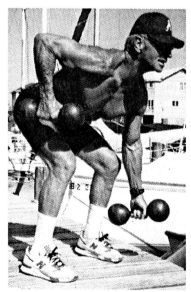

Bent Fly
Knees bent. Back straight. Slight bend in elbows. Lift weight above back.

(Upperback)

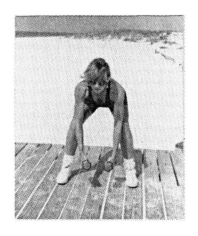 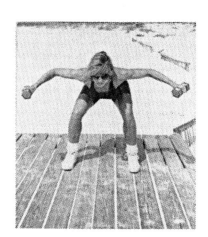

Pull Down
Alternate pulling weight to back and front
(Top and side of back. Arm and upper back)

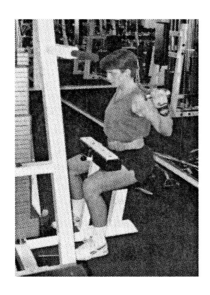 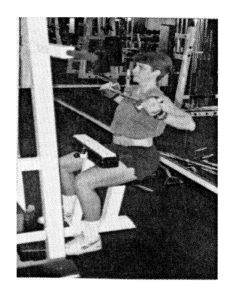

Dead Lift

Opposing grip on bar. Back straight. Slight bend in knees. Lift to standing position.
(Lower back and back of upper thigh)

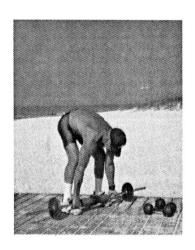
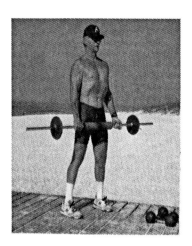

Back Extension

Slight bend in knees. Straighten back to horizontal.
(Lower back, buttocks and back of upper thigh)

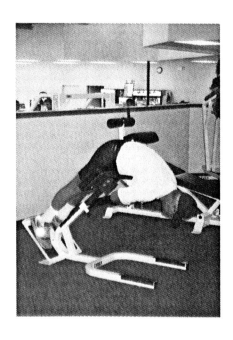
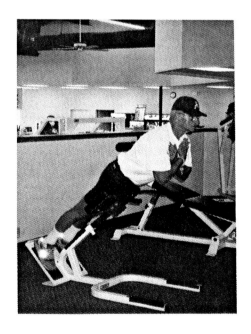

Chest
Bench Press
Two or alternate arms
Back flat on bench. Do not bounce weight on chest when lowering.
(Middle chest and back of upper arms)

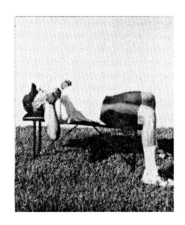 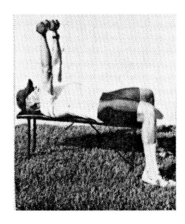 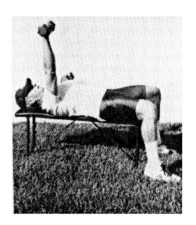

Bench Fly
Slight bend in arms. Lower to floor. Maintain arm bend
And raise to starting position.

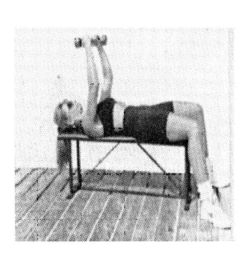 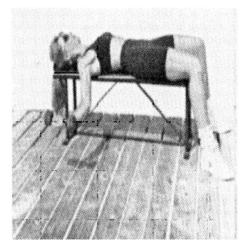

Arms
Biceps Curl
Two or alternate arms.
Elbows stabilized at sides. Full extension and flexion.
(Front of upper arm)

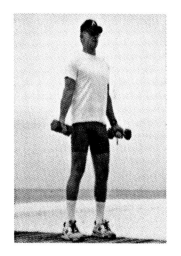 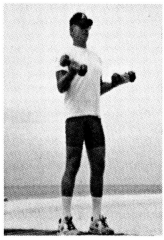 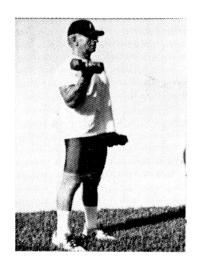

Triceps Overhead Extension
Elbow vertical. Lower all the way and then to full extension.
(Back of upper arm)

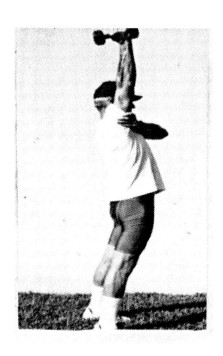 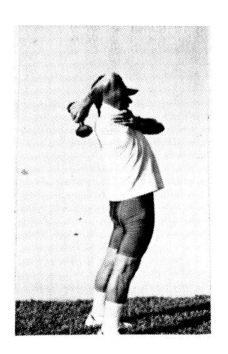

Triceps Extension
Upper arm parallel to floor. Fully extend.
(Back of upper arm)

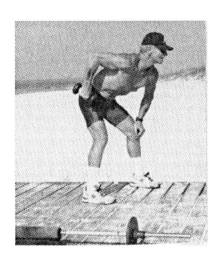 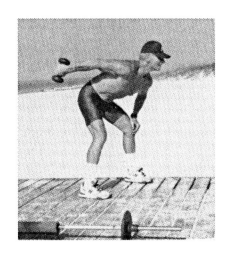

Dips
Lower body so that elbows are above shoulders. Extend.
(Back of upper arm. Chest and shoulders)

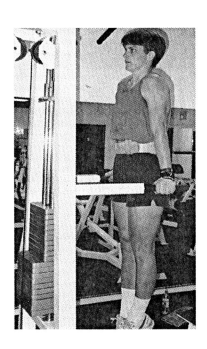 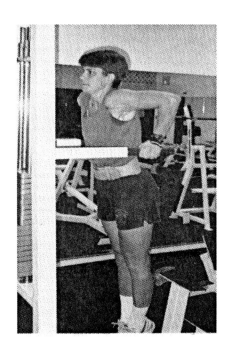

11

TRAINING PROGRAMS AND RECORDS

On the following pages are the program exercises, the number of reps and sets, their frequency, time between sets, method of lift and charts for keeping weight records.

Basic Conditioning Program

This program can be used for gains in strength (power) and body sculpting at a level which is suitable for those of us who are not specialists and are not striving to be competitive at an advanced level. It can precede the Performance Program and also be used as a maintenance program.

PERFORMANCE TRAINING

Performance Training utilizes multijoint/large muscle exercises. It is recommended for sports training, increasing speed, coordination, flexibility and for body weight control programs as well as developing functional strength. Performance Training may be the best single program for achieving these results. Advanced Body Sculpting requires a different approach.

Strength (Power) Training

Strength (Power) Training is for increasing the ability to lift heavy weights in multijoint movements often for competitive purposes.

Circuit Training

Circuit Training is for increasing endurance in addition to body sculpting and strength. It can be used in body weight control programs.

Body Sculpting (Body Building)

Body Sculpting is designed to alter the muscles for changing the body's shape.

Pre-Fatigue and Exhaust

Optional

A high intensity program for maximum muscle stimulation in a short period of time. It can be used as a program by itself, after the Basic Conditioning or following the preparation phase of Body Sculpting.

NOTE: There is evidence suggesting that a split program in Body Sculpting, Strength Training and Conditioning can be beneficial. A split program is dividing the day's exercises into two workouts. It could be done in the morning and evening, or as close as 30 minutes apart. Personal preference and time constraints may determine if a split program is for you.

BASIC CONDITIONING PROGRAM

This program is designed to increase strength, performance and improve body configuration for those of us who are less than Olympic caliber.

Phase I

Four Weeks

End Point	Elicit Fatigue
Reps	10
Sets	1
Lift Speed	Moderate
Frequency	3 Days / Week

* W - O - W - O - W

4 Days Active Rest

* W = Work Day, O = Off Day

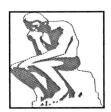

CONDITIONING PROGRAM
Phase I

Exercises	Reps	Date / Weight											
Back Squats	10												
Toe Raises	10												
Crunch Sit Ups	10												
Bent Row	10												
Bench Press	10												
Pull Lift	10												
Over Head Press	10												
Triceps OverH.	10												
Biceps Curl	10												
Shrugs	10												

Four Days Active Rest

Basic Conditioning Program

Phase II
Four Weeks

End Point	Elicit Fatigue
Reps	10
Sets	2
Lift Speed	Moderate
Time between sets	1-3 minutes
Frequency	3 Days/Week

W-O-W-O-W

Four Days Active Rest

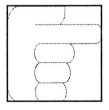

CONDITIONING PROGRAM

Phase II

Date

Exercises	Sets> Reps	1	2	1	2	1	2	1	2	1	2	1	2
		Weight											
Back Squats	10												
Toe Raises	10												
Crunch Sit Ups	10												
Bent Row	10												
Bench Press	10												
Pull Lift	10												
Over Head Press	10												
Triceps OverH.	10												
Biceps Curl	10												
Shrugs	10												

CONDITIONING PROGRAM

Phase II

Date

Exercises	Sets> Reps	1	2	1	2	1	2	1	2	1	2	1	2
		Weight											
Back Squats	10												
Toe Raises	10												
Crunch Sit Ups	10												
Bent Row	10												
Bench Press	10												
Pull Lift	10												
Over Head Press	10												
Triceps OverH.	10												
Biceps Curl	10												
Shrugs	10												

Five Days Active Rest

Basic Conditioning Program

Phase Three

Four Weeks

End Point	Elicit Fatigue
Reps	10
Sets	3
Speed	Moderate
Time between sets	1-3 minutes
Frequency	3 Days / Week

W - O - W - O - W
One Week Active Rest

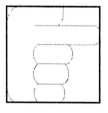

CONDITIONING PROGRAM
Phase III

		Date											
	Sets>	1	2	3	1	2	3	1	2	3	1	2	3
Exercises	Reps	Weight											
Back Squats	10												
Toe Raises	10												
Back Ext.	10												
Crunch Sit Ups	10												
OverH. Press	10												
Bent Row	10												
Pull Lift	10												
Triceps OverH.	10												
Biceps Curl	10												
Shrugs	10												

CONDITIONING PROGRAM
Phase III

		Date											
	Sets>	1	2	3	1	2	3	1	2	3	1	2	3
Exercises	Reps	Weight											
Back Squats	10												
Toe Raises	10												
Crunch Sit Ups	10												
OverH. Press	10												
Bent Row	10												
Bench Press	10												
Pull Lift	10												
Triceps OverH.	10												
Biceps Curl	10												
Shrugs	10												

CONDITIONING PROGRAM
Phase III

Date

Exercises	Sets>	1	2	3	1	2	3	1	2	3	1	2	3
	Reps	Weight											
Back Squats	10												
Toe Raises	10												
Snatch	8												
Crunch Sit Ups	10												
OverH. Press	10												
Bent Row	10												
Bench Press	10												
Pull Lift	10												
Triceps OverH.	10												
Biceps Curl	10												
Shrugs	10												

Five Days Active Rest

Begin New Cycle With Phase II

PERFORMANCE TRAINING

MULTIJOINT/LARGE MUSCLES

Preparation Phase 1

Two Weeks

The Preparation Phase is for developing proper technique as well as functional strength, and utilizes assistive exercises.

End Point	Heavy enough for resistance but light enough for learning technique.
Reps	8-10
Sets	1
Speed	Moderate
Frequency	Three days/week

W - O - W - O - W

Performance Training

Phase 1

Two Weeks

Date

Exercises	Reps	Weight					
Front Squat	10						
Back Squat	10						
Dead Lift	10						
Overhead Press	10						
Bent Row	10						
Pull Lift	10						
Push Jerk	10						

PERFORMANCE TRAINING

MULTIJOINT/LARGE MUSCLES

Preparation
Phase 2

Four Weeks

End Point	Heavy enough for resistance but light enough for learning technique.
Reps	8-10
Sets	1 for Two Weeks 2 for Two Weeks
Speed	Moderate
Time between sets	2-5 minutes
Frequency	Three days/week

W - O - W - O - W

Performance Training

Phase 2

Two Weeks

Date

Exercises	Reps	Weight					
Stretch Squat	10						
Lunge Squat	10						
Pull Lift	10						
Dead Lift	10						
Bent Row	10						
Jerk Split or Push	10						
Power Snatch	8						

Performance Training

Phase 2

Two Weeks

Date

Exercises	Sets Reps	1	2	1	2	1	2	1	2	1	2	1	2
		\multicolumn{12}{c}{Weight}												
Stretch Sq.													
Lunge Sq.													
Pull Lift													
Dead Lift													
Bent Row													
Split Jerk													
Snatch													

PERFORMANCE TRAINING

MULTIJOINT/LARGE MUSCLES

Preparation Phase 3

Three Weeks

End Point	Week 1: Heavy enough to elicit fatigue on last rep. Week 2: Heavy enough to elicit fatigue on last rep of each set. Week 3: Heavy enough for muscle failure on last rep of each set.
Reps	6-10
Sets	1 for First Week 2 for Second Week 3 for Third Week
Speed	Fast Concentric, Moderate
Time between sets	2-5 minutes
Frequency	Three days/week

W - O - W - O - W

Note: The Jerk part of the Clean and Jerk may be the front split, side split or push.

Performance Training
Phase 3

Week 1

Exercises	Reps	Date		
		Weight		
Bent Row	10			
Dead Lift	8			
Clean	8			
Clean & Jerkk	8			
Snatch	8			

Week 2

Exercises	Sets	Date					
		1	2	1	2	1	2
	Reps	Weight					
Bent Row	8						
Dead Lift	6						
Clean	8						
Clean & Jerk	6						
Snatch	8						

Week 3

Date

Exercises	Sets Reps	Weight								
Bent Row	10									
Dead Lift	8									
Clean	8									
Clean & Jerk	8									
Snatch	8									

Five Days Active Rest

PRE-FATIGUE AND EXHAUST
(Optional)

Two Weeks

The paired exercises should be done without a rest between them.

Point End	Heavy enough to elicit
Reps	10
Sets	1
Speed	Moderate
Frequency	Three days/week

W - O - W - O - W

PRE-FATIGUE AND EXHAUST
(Optional)

Two Weeks

Date

Exercises	Reps	Weight					
Leg Ext Squats	10						
Lateral Fly Overh. Press	10						
Shrugs Pull Lift	10						
Bench Press Bench Fly	10						
Bent Row Bent Fly	10						
Pulldown Biceps Curl	10						

CIRCUIT TRAINING

End Point	Heavy enough to elicit fatigue on last rep.
Reps	Moderate (10 reps)
	Advanced (15 reps)
Sets	2 Weeks, 1 Circuit
	3 Weeks, 2 Circuits
	2 Weeks, 3 Circuits
Frequency	3 Days/Week

Remember The Rules

1. Perform each exercise as rapidly as possible.

2. The final repetition should elicit fatigue.

3. a. When training for short-duration power events, make the transition from one exercise to the next as

    rapidly as possible.

   b. When training for endurance power events, allow no

    more than 60 seconds between exercises.

4. Train for as many as 3 circuits.

5. Keep a record of circuit times.

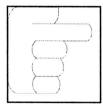

CIRCUIT TRAINING
One Circuit

Exercises	Reps 10/15	Weight					
		Date					
Toe Raises							
Back Squats							
Leg Curls							
Crunch Sit Ups							
Bent Row							
Overh. Press							
Clean & Jerk							
Bench Press							
Pull Ups							
Bench Fly							
Dips (men)							
Basket Hang (W)							
Biceps Curl							
Snatch	6						

Circuit Time						

CIRCUIT TRAINING
Two Circuits

		\multicolumn{10}{c}{Date}									
	Cir.>	1	2	1	2	1	2	1	2	1	2
Exercises	Reps 10/15	\multicolumn{10}{c}{Weight}									
Toe Raises											
Back Squat											
Leg Curls											
Crunch Sit Ups											
Bent Row											
Overh. Press											
Clean & Jerk											
Bench Press											
Bench Fly											
Dips (M)											
Basket Hang (W)											
Pull Downs											
Biceps Curls											
Snatch	6										

Circuit Time										
Total Time										

CIRCUIT TRAINING
Two Circuits

Exercises	Cir.> Reps 10/15	\multicolumn{10}{c}{Date / Weight}										
		1	2	1	2	1	2	1	2	1	2
Toe Raises											
Back Squat											
Leg Curls											
Crunch Sit Ups											
Bent Row											
Overh. Press											
Clean & Jerk											
Bench Press											
Bench Fly											
Dips (M)											
Basket Hang (W)											
Pull Downs											
Biceps Curls											
Snatch	6										
Circuit Time											
Total Time											

CIRCUIT TRAINING
Three Circuits

Date

Exercises	Circ.> Reps 10/15	1	2	3	1	2	3	1	2	3
		\multicolumn{9}{c}{Weight}									
Toe Raises										
Back Squat										
Leg Curls										
Crunch Sit Ups										
Bent Row										
Overh. Press										
Clean & Jerk										
Bench Press										
Bench Fly										
Dips (M)										
Basket Hang (W)										
Pull Downs										
Biceps Curls										
Snatch	6									

Circuit Time									
Total Time									

CIRCUIT TRAINING
Three Circuits

Date

Exercises	Reps 10/15	Circ.> 1	2	3	1	2	3	1	2	3
		\multicolumn{9}{c}{Weight}								
Toe Raises										
Back Squat										
Leg Curls										
Crunch Sit Ups										
Bent Row										
Overh. Press										
Clean & Jerk										
Bench Press										
Bench Fly										
Dips (M)										
Basket Hang (W)										
Pull Downs										
Biceps Curls										
Snatch	6									

Circuit Time									
Total Time									

Body Sculpting (Body Building)

Programs	
<u>Moderate</u>	<u>Advanced</u>
Phases:	Phases:
Preparation	Volume
Volume	Advanced Volume
Peak	Intensity
	Peak
	Preparation Phase
	Two - Four Weeks
End Point	Weight heavy enough to elicit fatigue on last rep.
Reps	10
Sets	1
Speed	Moderate
Frequency	Three days/week

W - O - W - O - W

Five Days Active Rest

Stretching

Light Aerobics

Low Intensity Calisthenics

BODY SCULPTING
Preparation Phase

Date

Exercises	Reps	Weight										
Back Squats	10											
Overh. Press	10											
Bent Row	10											
Bench Press	10											
Pull Lift	10											
Lateral Fly	10											
Bent Fly	10											
Tric. Overh.	10											
Biceps Curl	10											
Crunches	15											

Five Days Active Rest

BODY SCULPTING

Volume Phase
Four Weeks

End Point	Weight heavy enough to elicit fatigue on last rep each set.
Reps	12
Sets	4
Speed	2 wks. Slow Con. & Ecc.
	2 wks. Mod. Con. & Slow Ecc.
Time between sets	1-2 minutes
Frequency	4 Days / Week

W - W - O - W - W

Five Days Active Rest

BODY SCULPTING
Volume Phase

Day #1 _____

Day #1

Exercises	Reps	Sets 1	2	3	4
			Weight		
Back Squats	12				
Toe Raises	12				
Leg Curl	12				
Leg Ext.	12				
Back Ext.	12		XXX		XXX
Crunches	15				
Pulldown	12				

Day #2 _____

Exercises	Reps	Sets 1	2	3	4
			Weight		
Bench Press	12				
Bench Fly	12				
Lateral Fly	12				
Pull Lift	12				
Overh. Press	12				
Biceps Curl	12				
Tric. Overh.	12				

Day #3 _____

Exercises	Reps	Sets 1	2	3	4
			Weight		
Back Squats	12				
Toe Raises	12				
Leg Curl	12				
Leg Ext.	12				
Back Ext.	12		XXX		XXX
Crunches	15				
Pulldown	12				

Day #4 _____

Exercises	Reps	Sets 1	2	3	4
			Weight		
Bench Press	12				
Bench Fly	12				
Lateral Fly	12				
Pull Lift	12				
Overh. Press	12				
Biceps Curl	12				
Tric. Overh.	12				

BODY SCULPTING
Volume Phase

Day #5 _____

Exercises	Reps	Sets 1	2	3	4
			Weight		
Back Squats	12				
Toe Raises	12				
Leg Curl	12				
Leg Ext.	12				
Back Ext.	12		XXX		XXX
Crunches	15				
Pulldown	12				

Day #6 _____

Exercises	Reps	Sets 1	2	3	4
			Weight		
Bench Press	12				
Bench Fly	12				
Lateral Fly	12				
Pull Lift	12				
Overh. Press	12				
Biceps Curl	12				
Tric. Overh.	12				

Day #7 _____

Exercises	Reps	Sets 1	2	3	4
			Weight		
Back Squats	12				
Toe Raises	12				
Leg Curl	12				
Leg Ext.	12				
Back Ext.	12		XXX		XXX
Crunches	15				
Pulldown	12				

Day #8 _____

Exercises	Reps	Sets 1	2	3	4
			Weight		
Bench Press	12				
Bench Fly	12				
Lateral Fly	12				
Pull Lift	12				
Overh. Press	12				
Biceps Curl	12				
Tric. Overh.	12				

BODY SCULPTING
Volume Phase

Day #9 _____

Exercises	Reps	Sets 1	2	3	4
			Weight		
Back Squats	12				
Toe Raises	12				
Leg Curl	12				
Leg Ext.	12				
Back Ext.	12		XXX		XXX
Crunches	15				
Pulldown	12				

Day #10 _____

Exercises	Reps	Sets 1	2	3	4
			Weight		
Bench Press	12				
Bench Fly	12				
Lateral Fly	12				
Pull Lift	12				
Overh. Press	12				
Biceps Curl	12				
Tric. Overh.	12				

Day #11 _____

Exercises	Reps	Sets 1	2	3	4
			Weight		
Back Squats	12				
Toe Raises	12				
Leg Curl	12				
Leg Ext.	12				
Back Ext.	12		XXX		XXX
Crunches	15				
Pulldown	12				

Day #12 _____

Exercises	Reps	Sets 1	2	3	4
			Weight		
Bench Press	12				
Bench Fly	12				
Lateral Fly	12				
Pull Lift	12				
Overh. Press	12				
Biceps Curl	12				
Tric. Overh.	12				

BODY SCULPTING
Volume Phase

Day #13 _____

Exercises	Reps	\multicolumn{4}{c}{Sets}			
		1	2	3	4
		\multicolumn{4}{c}{Weight}			
Front Squats	12				
Toe Raises	12				
Leg Curl	12				
Leg Ext.	12				
Back Ext.	12		XXX		XXX
Crunches	15				
Pulldown	12				

Day #14 _____

Exercises	Reps	\multicolumn{4}{c}{Sets}			
		1	2	3	4
		\multicolumn{4}{c}{Weight}			
Bench Press	12				
Bench Fly	12				
Lateral Fly	12				
Pull Lift	12				
Overh. Press	12				
Biceps Curl	12				
Tric. Overh.	12				

Day #15 _____

Exercises	Reps	\multicolumn{4}{c}{Sets}			
		1	2	3	4
		\multicolumn{4}{c}{Weight}			
Front Squats	12				
Toe Raises	12				
Leg Curl	12				
Leg Ext.	12				
Back Ext.	12		XXX		XXX
Crunches	15				
Pulldown	12				

Day #16 _____

Exercises	Reps	\multicolumn{4}{c}{Sets}			
		1	2	3	4
		\multicolumn{4}{c}{Weight}			
Bench Press	12				
Bench Fly	12				
Lateral Fly	12				
Pull Lift	12				
Overh. Press	12				
Biceps Curl	12				
Tric. Overh.	12				

Five Days Active Rest

BODY SCULPTING

Advanced Volume Phase

Four Weeks

End Point	Weight heavy enough to elicit fatigue on last rep of each set.
Reps	12
Sets	4
Speed	2 wks. Slow Con. & Ecc. 2 wks. Mod. Con. & Slow Ecc.
Time between sets	1-2 minutes
Frequency	6 Days / Week

W - W - O - W - W

One Week Active Rest

BODY SCULPTING
Advanced Volume Phase

Day #1 _____

		Sets			
		1	2	3	4
Exercises	Reps	Weight			
Back Squats	12				
Toe Raises	12				
Leg Curl	12				
Leg Ext.	12				
Crunches	15				
Biceps Curl	12				
Tric. Overh.	12				

Day #2 _____

		Sets			
		1	2	3	4
Exercises	Reps	Weight			
Bench Press	12				
Basket Hang	12				
Bench Fly	12				
Overh. Press	12				
Pull Lift	12				
Shrugs	12				

Day # 3 _____

		Sets			
		1	2	3	4
Exercises	Reps	Weight			
Pulldown	12				
Bent Fly	12				
Lateral Fly	12				
Dips	10				
Bent Row	12				

Day #4 _____

		Sets			
		1	2	3	4
Exercises	Reps	Weight			
Back Squats	12				
Toe Raises	12				
Leg Curl	12				
Leg Ext.	12				
Crunches	12				
Biceps Curl	12				
Tric. Overh.	12				

BODY SCULPTING
Advanced Volume Phase

Day # 5 _____

Exercises	Reps	Sets 1	2	3	4
		Weight			
Bench Press	12				
Basket Hang	10				
Bench Fly	12				
Overh. Press	12				
Pull Lift	12				
Shrugs	20				

Day #6 _____

Exercises	Reps	Sets 1	2	3	4
		Weight			
Pulldowns	12				
Bent Fly	12				
Lateral Fly	12				
Dips	10				
Bent Row	12				

Day #7 _____

Exercises	Reps	Sets 1	2	3	4
		Weight			
Front Squats	12				
Toe Raises	12				
Leg Curl	12				
Leg Ext.	12				
Crunches	15				
Biceps Curl	12				
Tric. Overh.	12				

Day #8 _____

Exercises	Reps	Sets 1	2	3	4
		Weight			
Bench Press	12				
Basket Hang	10				
Bench Fly	12				
Overh. Press	12				
Pull Lift	12				
Shrugs	12				

BODY SCULPTING
Advanced Volume Phase

Day # 9 _____

Sets

Exercises	Reps	1	2	3	4
		Weight			
Pulldown	12				
Bent Fly	12				
Lateral Fly	12				
Dips	10				
Bent Row	12				

Day #10 _____

Sets

Exercises	Reps	1	2	3	4
		Weight			
Back Squats	12				
Toe Raises	12				
Leg Curl	12				
Leg Ext.	12				
Crunches	15				
Biceps Curl	12				
Tric. Overh.	12				

Day # 11 _____

Sets

Exercises	Reps	1	2	3	4
		Weight			
Bench Press	12				
Basket Hang	10				
Bench Fly	12				
Overh. Press	12				
Pull Lift	12				
Shrugs	20				

Day #12 _____

Sets

Exercises	Reps	1	2	3	4
		Weight			
Pulldowns	12				
Bent Fly	12				
Lateral Fly	12				
Dips	10				
Bent Row	12				

BODY SCULPTING
Advanced Volume Phase

Day #13 _____

Exercises	Reps	Sets 1	2	3	4
		Weight			
Front Squats	12				
Toe Raises	12				
Leg Curl	12				
Leg Ext.	12				
Crunches	15				
Biceps Curl	12				
Tric. Overh.	12				

Day #14 _____

Exercises	Reps	Sets 1	2	3	4
		Weight			
Bench Press	12				
Basket Hang	12				
Bench Fly	12				
Overh. Press	12				
Pull Lift	12				

Day #15 _____

Exercises	Reps	Sets 1	2	3	4
		Weight			
Pulldown	12				
Bent Fly	12				
Lateral Fly	12				
Dips	10				
Bent Row	12				

Day #16 _____

Exercises	Reps	Sets 1	2	3	4
		Weight			
Front Squats	12				
Toe Raises	12				
Leg Curl	12				
Leg Ext.	12				
Crunches	15				
Biceps Curl	12				
Tric. Overh.	12				

BODY SCULPTING
Advanced Volume Phase

Day #17 _____

		Sets			
		1	2	3	4
Exercises	Reps	Weight			
Bench Press	12				
Basket Hang	10				
Bench Fly	12				
Overh. Press	12				
Pull Lift	12				
Shrugs	20				

Day #18 _____

		Sets			
		1	2	3	4
Exercises	Reps	Weight			
Pulldowns	12				
Bent Fly	12				
Lateral Fly	12				
Dips	10				
Bent Row	12				

Day #19 _____

		Sets			
		1	2	3	4
Exercises	Reps	Weight			
Front Squats	12				
Toe Raises	12				
Leg Curl	12				
Leg Ext.	12				
Crunches	15				
Biceps Curl	12				
Tric. Overh.	12				

Day #20 _____

		Sets			
		1	2	3	4
Exercises	Reps	Weight			
Bench Press	12				
Basket Hang	10				
Bench Fly	12				
Overh. Press	12				
Pull Lift	12				
Shrugs	12				

BODY SCULPTING
Advanced Volume Phase

Day #21 _____

Exercises	Reps	\multicolumn{4}{c}{Sets}			
		1	2	3	4
		\multicolumn{4}{c}{Weight}			
Pulldown	12				
Bent Fly	12				
Lateral Fly	12				
Dips	10				
Bent Row	12				

Day #22 _____

Exercises	Reps	Sets			
		1	2	3	4
		Weight			
Front Squats	12				
Toe Raises	12				
Leg Curl	12				
Leg Ext.	12				
Crunches	15				
Biceps Curl	12				
Tric. Overh.	12				

Day #21 _____

Exercises	Reps	Sets			
		1	2	3	4
		Weight			
Bench Press	12				
Basket Hang	10				
Bench Fly	12				
Overh. Press	12				
Pull Lift	12				
Shrugs	20				

Day #22 _____

Exercises	Reps	Sets			
		1	2	3	4
		Weight			
Pulldowns	12				
Bent Fly	12				
Lateral Fly	12				
Dips	10				
Bent Row	12				

One Week Active Rest

BODY SCULPTING

Intensity Phase

Four Weeks

End Point	Weight heavy enough to elicit fatigue on last rep of first two sets and max muscle failure on last rep of third set.
Reps	8
Sets	3
Speed	2 wks. Mod. Con. & Ecc. 2 wks. Mod. Con. & Slow Ecc.
Time between sets	1-2 minutes
Frequency	4 Days / Week

W - W - O - W - W

Five Days Active Rest

BODY SCULPTING
Intensity Phase

Day #1 _____

Exercises	Reps	Sets 1	2	3
		Weight		
Back Squats	8			
Toe Raises	8			
Leg Curl	8			
Leg Ext.	8			
Crunch Sit Ups	15			
Basket Hang	8			
Biceps Curl	8			
Tric. Overh.	8			
Triceps Ext.	8			

Day #2 _____

Exercises	Reps	Sets 1	2	3
		Weight		
Overh. Press	8			
Bent Row	8			
Bench Press	8			
Pull Lift	8			
Bench Fly	8			
Pulldown	8			
Dips	12			
Lateral Fly	8			
Shrugs	8			
Snatch	8			

BODY SCULPTING
Intensity Phase

Day #3 _____

Exercises	Reps	Sets 1	2	3
			Weight	
Back Squats	8			
Toe Raises	8			
Leg Curl	8			
Leg Ext.	8			
Crunch Sit Ups	15			
Basket Hang	8			
Biceps Curl	8			
Tric. Overh.	8			
Triceps Ext.	8			

Day #4 _____

Exercises	Reps	Sets 1	2	3
			Weight	
Overh. Press	8			
Bent Row	8			
Bench Press	8			
Pull Lift	8			
Bench Fly	8			
Pulldown	8			
Dips	12			
Lateral Fly	8			
Shrugs	8			
Snatch	8			XXX

BODY SCULPTING
Intensity Phase

Day #5 _____   Day #6 _____

Exercises	Reps	Sets Weight		
		1	2	3
Back Squats	8			
Toe Raises	8			
Leg Curl	8			
Leg Ext.	8			
Crunch Sit Ups	10			
Basket Hang	8			
Biceps Curl	8			
Tric. Overh.	8			
Triceps Ext.	8			

Exercises	Reps	Sets Weight		
		1	2	3
Overh. Press	8			
Bent Row	8			
Bench Press	8			
Pull Lift	8			
Bench Fly	8			
Pulldown	8			
Dips	MAX			
Lateral Fly	8			
Shrugs	8			
Snatch	8			XXX

BODY SCULPTING
Intensity Phase

Day #7 _____

Exercises	Reps	Sets 1	2	3
		Weight		
Front Squats	8			
Toe Raises	8			
Leg Curl	8			
Leg Ext.	8			
Crunch Sit Ups	10			
Basket Hang	8			
Biceps Curl	8			
Tric. Overh.	8			
Triceps Ext.	8			

Day #8 _____

Exercises	Reps	Sets 1	2	3
		Weight		
Overh. Press	8			
Bent Row	8			
Bench Press	8			
Pull Lift	8			
Bench Fly	8			
Pulldown	8			
Dips	10			
Lateral Fly	8			
Shrugs	8			
Snatch	8			XXX

BODY SCULPTING
Intensity Phase

Day #9 _____   Day #10 _____

Day #9

Exercises	Reps	Sets 1	2	3
		Weight		
Front Squats	8			
Toe Raises	8			
Leg Curl	8			
Leg Ext.	8			
Crunch Sit Ups	12			
Basket Hang	8			
Biceps Curl	8			
Tric. Overh.	8			
Triceps Ext.	8			

Day #10

Exercises	Reps	Sets 1	2	3
		Weight		
Overh. Press	8			
Bent Row	8			
Bench Press	8			
Pull Lift	8			
Bench Fly	8			
Pulldown	8			
Dips	MAX			
Lateral Fly	8			
Shrugs	8			
Snatch	8			XXX

BODY SCULPTING
Intensity Phase

Day #11 _____

Exercises	Reps	Sets 1	2	3
			Weight	
Front Squats	8			
Toe Raises	8			
Leg Curl	8			
Leg Ext.	8			
Crunch Sit Ups	12			
Basket Hang	8			
Biceps Curl	8			
Tric. Overh.	8			
Triceps Ext.	8			

Day #12 _____

Exercises	Reps	Sets 1	2	3
			Weight	
Overh. Press	8			
Bent Row	8			
Bench Press	8			
Pull Lift	8			
Bench Fly	8			
Pulldown	8			
Dips	10			
Lateral Fly	8			
Shrugs	8			
Snatch	8			XXX

BODY SCULPTING
Intensity Phase

Day #13 _____

		Sets		
		1	2	3
Exercises	Reps	Weight		
Front Squats	8			
Toe Raises	8			
Leg Curl	8			
Leg Ext.	8			
Crunch Sit Ups	10			
Basket Hang	8			
Biceps Curl	8			
Tric. Overh.	8			
Triceps Ext.	8			

Day #14 _____

		Sets		
		1	2	3
Exercises	Reps	Weight		
Overh. Press	8			
Bent Row	8			
Bench Press	8			
Pull Lift	8			
Bench Fly	8			
Pulldown	8			
Dips	10			
Lateral Fly	8			
Shrugs	8			
Snatch	8			XXX

BODY SCULPTING
Intensity Phase

Day #15 _____

Exercises	Reps	Sets 1	2	3
		Weight		
Front Squats	8			
Toe Raises	8			
Leg Curl	8			
Leg Ext.	8			
Crunch Sit Ups	10			
Basket Hang	8			
Biceps Curl	8			
Tric. Overh.	8			
Triceps Ext.	8			

Day #16 _____

Exercises	Reps	Sets 1	2	3
		Weight		
Overh. Press	8			
Bent Row	8			
Bench Press	8			
Pull Lift	8			
Bench Fly	8			
Pulldown	8			
Dips	10			
Lateral Fly	8			
Shrugs	8			
Snatch	8			XXX

Five Days Active Rest

BODY SCULPTING

Peak Phase

Two Weeks

End Point	Weight heavy enough to elicit fatigue on last rep of first set and max muscle failure on last rep of third set.
Reps	3
Sets	3
Speed	Moderate
Time between sets	1-2 minutes
Frequency	3 Days / Week

W - W - O - W - W

Five Days Active Rest

BODY SCULPTING
Peak Phase

		\multicolumn{3}{c}{Date}						

Exercises	Sets>	1	2	3	1	2	3	1	2	3
	Reps				Weight					
Back Squats	3									
Toe Raises	3									
Leg Curl	3									
Leg Ext.	3									
Crunch Sit Ups	15									
Overh. Press	3									
Bent Row	3									
Bench Press										
Pull Lift	3									
Pulldown	3									
Dips	MAX									
Biceps Curl	3									
Triceps Overh.	3									
Snatch	3									

BODY SCULPTING
Peak Phase

Date

Exercises	Sets>	1	2	3	1	2	3	1	2	3
	Reps	Weight								
Back Squats	3									
Toe Raises	3									
Leg Curl	3									
Leg Ext.	3									
Crunch Sit Ups	15									
Overh. Press	3									
Bent Row	3									
Bench Press										
Pull Lift	3									
Pulldown	3									
Dips	MAX									
Biceps Curl	3									
Triceps Overh.	3									
Snatch	3									

Five Days Active Rest
Begin New Cycle With The Volume Phase

Strength (Power) Training

Preparation Phase

Two - Four Weeks

End Point	Weight heavy enough to elicit fatigue on the last rep.
Reps	10
Sets	1
Speed	Moderate
Frequency	3 Days / Week

W - O - W - O - W
Five Days Active Rest

Strength (POWER) Training
Preparation Phase

Date

Exercises	Reps	Weight											
Back Squats	10												
Toe Raises	10												
Crunch Sit Ups	15												
Dead Lift	10												
Overh. Press	10												
Bench Press	10												
Pull Lift	10												
Pulldown	10												
Dips	10												
Snatch	15												

Five Days Active Rest

STRENGTH (POWER) TRAINING
Volume Phase

Four Weeks

End Point	Weight heavy enough to elicit fatigue on last rep of first three sets and muscle failure on last set.
Reps	8
Sets	4
Speed	2 wks. Slow Con. & Ecc. 2 wks. Moderate.
Time between sets	2-4 minutes
Frequency	4 Days / Week

W - W - O - W - W

Five Days Active Rest

STRENGTH TRAINING
Volume Phase

Day #1_____

Sets

Exercises	Reps	1	2	3	4
		Weight			
Back Squats	8				
Leg Curl	8				
Leg Ext.	8				
Dips	15				
Dead Lift	8				
Crunches	15				

Day #2_____

Sets

Exercises	Reps	1	2	3	4
		Weight			
Bench Press	8				
Pull Lift	8				
Bent Row	8				
Overh. Press	8				
Snatch	8			XXX	XXX

Day #3_____

Sets

Exercises	Reps	1	2	3	4
		Weight			
Back Squats	8				
Leg Curl	8				
Leg Ext.	8				
Dips	15				
Dead Lift	8				
Crunches	15				

Day #4_____

Sets

Exercises	Reps	1	2	3	4
		Weight			
Bench Press	8				
Pull Lift	8				
Bent Row	8				
Overh. Press	8				
Snatch	8			XXX	XXX

STRENGTH TRAINING
Volume Phase

Day #5 _____

Sets

Exercises	Reps	1	2	3	4
		Weight			
Back Squats	8				
Leg Curl	8				
Leg Ext.	8				
Dips	MAX				
Dead Lift	8				
Crunches	15				

Day #6 _____

Sets

Exercises	Reps	1	2	3	4
		Weight			
Bench Press	8				
Pull Lift	8				
Bent Row	8				
Overh. Press	8				
Snatch	8			XXX	XXX

Day #7 _____

Sets

Exercises	Reps	1	2	3	4
		Weight			
Back Squats	8				
Leg Curl	8				
Leg Ext.	8				
Dips	MAX				
Dead Lift	8				
Crunches	15				

Day #8 _____

Sets

Exercises	Reps	1	2	3	4
		Weight			
Bench Press	8				
Pull Lift	8				
Bent Row	8				
Overh. Press	8				
Snatch	8			XXX	XXX

STRENGTH TRAINING
Volume Phase

Day #9 _____

Sets

Exercises	Reps	1	2	3	4
		Weight			
Back Squats	8				
Leg Curl	8				
Leg Ext.	8				
Dips	MAX				
Dead Lift	8				
Crunches	15				

Day #10 _____

Sets

Exercises	Reps	1	2	3	4
		Weight			
Bench Press	8				
Pull Lift	8				
Bent Row	8				
Overh. Press	8				
Snatch	8			XXX	XXX

Day #11 _____

Sets

Exercises	Reps	1	2	3	4
		Weight			
Back Squats	8				
Leg Curl	8				
Leg Ext.	8				
Dips	MAX				
Dead Lift	8				
Crunches	15				

Day #12 _____

Sets

Exercises	Reps	1	2	3	4
		Weight			
Bench Press	8				
Pull Lift	8				
Bent Row	8				
Overh. Press	8				
Snatch	8			XXX	XXX

STRENGTH TRAINING
Volume Phase

Day #13 _____

Sets

Exercises	Reps	1	2	3	4
		Weight			
Back Squats	8				
Leg Curl	8				
Leg Ext.	8				
Dips	MAX				
Dead Lift	8				
Crunches	15				

Day #14 _____

Sets

Exercises	Reps	1	2	3	4
		Weight			
Bench Press	8				
Pull Lift	8				
Bent Row	8				
Overh. Press	8				
Snatch	8			XXX	XXX

Day #15 _____

Sets

Exercises	Reps	1	2	3	4
		Weight			
Back Squats	8				
Leg Curl	8				
Leg Ext.	8				
Dips	MAX				
Dead Lift	8				
Crunches	15				

Day #16 _____

Sets

Exercises	Reps	1	2	3	4
		Weight			
Bench Press	8				
Pull Lift	8				
Bent Row	8				
Overh. Press	8				
Snatch	8				XXX

Five Days Active Rest

STRENGTH (POWER) TRAINING
Intensity Phase

Three Weeks

End Point	Weight heavy enough to elicit fatigue on last rep of first set and max muscle failure on last rep of the last two sets.
NOTE:	The Intensity and Peak Phases may be enhanced by doing each repetition at the maximum weight which can be lifted one time. This means hanging to a lower weight on each rep until the indicated number in the set has been achieved.
Reps	6
Sets	3
Speed	Moderate
Time between sets	2-4 minutes
Frequency	4 Days / Week

W - W - O - W - W

5 Days Active Rest

STRENGTH (Power) PHASE
Intensity Phase

Day #1 _____

		Sets 1	2	3	4
Exercises	Reps	Weight			
Back Squats	6				
Leg Curl	6				
Leg Ext.	6				
Dips	MAX				
Dead Lift	6				
Crunches	15				

Day #2 _____

		Sets 1	2	3	4
Exercises	Reps	Weight			
Bench Press	6				
Pull Lift	6				
Bent Row	6				
Overh. Press	6				
Snatch	6				XXX

Day #3 _____

		Sets 1	2	3	4
Exercises	Reps	Weight			
Back Squats	6				
Leg Curl	6				
Leg Ext.	6				
Dips	MAX				
Dead Lift	6				
Crunches	15				

Day #4 _____

		Sets 1	2	3	4
Exercises	Reps	Weight			
Bench Press	6				
Pull Lift	6				
Bent Row	6				
Overh. Press	6				
Snatch	6				XXX

STRENGTH TRAINING
Intensity Phase

Day #5 _____

Exercises	Reps	Sets 1	2	3	4
		Weight			
Back Squats	6				
Leg Curl	6				
Leg Ext.	6				
Dips	MAX				
Dead Lift	6				
Crunches	15				

Day #6 _____

Exercises	Reps	Sets 1	2	3	4
		Weight			
Bench Press	6				
Pull Lift	6				
Bent Row	6				
Overh. Press	6				
Snatch	6				XXX

Day #7 _____

Exercises	Reps	Sets 1	2	3	4
		Weight			
Back Squats	6				
Leg Curl	6				
Leg Ext.	6				
Dips	MAX				
Dead Lift	6				
Crunches	15				

Day #8 _____

Exercises	Reps	Sets 1	2	3	4
		Weight			
Bench Press	6				
Pull Lift	6				
Bent Row	6				
Overh. Press	6				
Snatch	6				XXX

STRENGTH TRAINING
Intensity Phase

Day #9 _____

Exercises	Reps	Sets 1	2	3	4
		Weight			
Back Squats	6				
Toe Raises	6				
Leg Curl	6				
Leg Ext.	6				
Dips	MAX				
Crunches	15				
Dead Lift	6				

Day #10 _____

Exercises	Reps	Sets 1	2	3	4
		Weight			
Bench Press	6				
Pull Lift	6				
Bent Row	6				
Overh. Press	6				
Pulldown	6				
Snatch					XXX

Day #11 _____

Exercises	Reps	Sets 1	2	3	4
		Weight			
Back Squats	6				
Toe Raises	6				
Leg Curl	6				
Leg Ext.	6				
Dips	MAX				
Crunches	15				
Dead Lift	6				

Day #12 _____

Exercises	Reps	Sets 1	2	3	4
		Weight			
Bench Press	6				
Pull Lift	6				
Bent Row	6				
Overh. Press	6				
Pulldown	6				
Snatch					XXX

Five Days Active Rest

STRENGTH TRAINING
Peak Phase

Two Weeks

End Point	Max muscle failure on last rep of each set.
NOTE:	The Intensity and Peak Phases may be enhanced by doing each repetition at the maximum weight which can be lifted one time. This means changing to a lower weight on each rep until the indicated number in the set has been achieved.
Reps	3
Sets	2
Speed	Fast Con. & Ecc.
Time between sets	2-4 minutes
Frequency	3 Days / Week

W - W - O - W - W

Begin New Cycle With the Volume Phase

STRENGTH TRAINING
Peak Phase

Day #1 _____

Exercises	Reps	Sets 1 Weight	2
Front Squats	3		
Toe Raises	3		
Leg Curl	3		
Leg Ext.	3		
Crunch Sit Ups	15		
Dead Lift	3		
Dips	MAX		

Day #2 _____

Exercises	Reps	Sets 1 Weight	2
Overh. Press	3		
Bent Row	3		
Bench Press	3		
Pull Lift	3		
Pulldown	3		
Snatch	3		

Day #3 _____

Exercises	Reps	Sets 1 Weight	2
Front Squats	3		
Toe Raises	3		
Leg Curl	3		
Leg Ext.	3		
Crunch Sit Ups	15		
Dead Lift	3		
Dips	MAX		

Day #4 _____

Exercises	Reps	Sets 1 Weight	2
Overh. Press	3		
Bent Row	3		
Bench Press	3		
Pull Lift	3		
Pulldown	3		
Snatch	3		

STRENGTH TRAINING
Peak Phase

Day #5 _____

		Sets	
		1	2
Exercises	Reps	Weight	
Front Squats	3		
Toe Raises	3		
Leg Curl	3		
Leg Ext.	3		
Crunch Sit Ups	15		
Dead Lift	3		
Dips	MAX		

Day #6 _____

		Sets	
		1	2
Exercises	Reps	Weight	
Overh. Press	3		
Bent Row	3		
Bench Press	3		
Pull Lift	3		
Pulldown	3		
Snatch	3		

Day #7 _____

		Sets	
		1	2
Exercises	Reps	Weight	
Front Squats	3		
Toe Raises	3		
Leg Curl	3		
Leg Ext.	3		
Crunch Sit Ups	15		
Dead Lift	3		
Dips	MAX		

Day #8 _____

		Sets	
		1	2
Exercises	Reps	Weight	
Overh. Press	3		
Bent Row	3		
Bench Press	3		
Pull Lift	3		
Pulldown	3		
Snatch	3		

One Week Active Rest
Begin New Cycle With The Volume Phase

Additional Training Records

ORDER FORM

Please send an additional set of Training Records for:

                     Price

Conditioning	$2.00	_____
Performance Tr.	2.00	_____
Circuit Training	2.00	_____
Body Sculpting	3.00	_____
Strength Training	3.00	_____
Pre-Fatigue & Exhaust	2.00	_____
Total	$	_____
Shipping	$2.00	
Total	$	_____

Name_____

Address_____

City _____State_____Zip_____

    Mail Payment and Order Form To:

        Don McDaniel, Ed.D, CSCS, CPT
        1503 Rivers Street
        Pensacola, Fl 32514

        E-mail: mcd@pcola.gulf.net

PART 2
12
Eating Behavior
CORRECTING EATING MISBEHAVIOR

There is nothing more interesting to most of us than the broad subject of what and how to eat. As a result there are huge numbers of people and interest groups who are more than willing to supply just such information.

Unfortunately the vast majority of the information is uninformed, not backed by creditable data or just plain bunk and nonsense. Who knows the data? Not many. It is not often one can find people who have both the hard data and the analytical mind to use it.

In no way do I claim even a small amount of omnipotence about the subject. In fact each day I realize I know less and less. Not much longer and I'll be too ignorant to exist.

With that said, allow me to share with you current data as I understand it. Many of you will be disappointed in what you read. Do not look for detailed specifics as to what to do every day. Sounds good but it is not possible to correctly prescribe exactly what each individual should eat every meal every day. Intensive individual medical supervision may be the possible exception

For countless centuries our kind struggled to get enough to eat. It made little difference what it was, we were glad to get it. Much of the world is still that way. Now that we, most of us that is, have an over-abundance of food, we are told not to eat so much. The problem is that we seem to go from feast to famine or, in this case, from famine to feast, and, as with most things, we go to extremes.

In many ways we have come to feel guilty about eating, particularly if it tastes good. Eat something which tastes good and it is a mortal sin, or so it seems.

Forget the guilt. Eating should be a pleasure!

One can ponder why we have struggled so hard to improve our food technology to make things taste good only to be told that it's bad for us. If it's salty, greasy or sweet it may taste good, but, according to the so-called experts, beware of the results.

For the past few decades, the race for the consumer dollar, improved refrigeration and transportation, better sanitation and good chemistry has given us unparalleled food quantity and quality. To not avail ourselves of these advances and enjoy them doesn't make sense.

To paraphrase, never in the history of human affairs has there been so much eating behavior misinformation, espoused and believed by so many, to the benefit of so few. Correct eating is not complicated. We have come to think that there are all sorts of weird combinations of what and how to eat. There are not. It seems that unless the instructions are exotic and new they aren't good. Unless the product or diet is made to sound revolutionary it has no appeal. Correct eating behavior is simple. There are no tricks. The basics are not new, although there is a "new" diet every week. New means new marketing, profits, and, too often, gullibility. If a book were written several thousand years ago about the facts of the biochemistry of human nutrition, it would read the same as it would today. The basics don't change, only the hype. Someone suggested there are more than 10,000 books on nutrition. If any one was the answer we would not need the other 9,999.

It is amazing how we forsake good sense when it comes to how we should eat!

To begin with there is no such thing as good food and bad food. I know of no food which will kill you if eaten occasionally, or a food which wouldn't be bad if it was the only food eaten for a prolonged period of time. True, there are some foods which should not be eaten in excessive amounts, but correct eating behavior is a matter of <u>balance</u>, <u>frequency</u> and <u>amount</u>.

Almost everyone wants to know exactly what to eat for each meal, when should it be eaten and how many calories should be consumed. In other words we want a specific, detailed diet and all the charts and lists which go with it. For the most part, such information, after a few weeks, is laid aside and forgotten.

No one follows a diet or counts calories for very long. It sounds great to say we are on a diet and enduring distasteful, no pun intended, restrictions, but after the martyr complex wears off it's goodbye to good intentions.

Not only do nutrition intentions go by the wayside, the information is soon forgotten or ignored.

It's impressive to concoct diets and publish lists. Maybe it sells books, but seldom does the information have a lasting impact.

What you will find here are the things which make sense and are understandable. If, occasionally, you wish to refer to lists and specifics, try the American Heart Association's books or a public school health education text. Better yet, if at any given time you think you need specifics consult with a Registered Dietician. They are the pros!

Another lesson learned the hard way is that no two people respond to food in exactly the same way. Individual tastes, absorption processes and metabolic rates are different. As a result, mass prescriptions make good copy and reading, but usually fall far short of being appropriate for the individual.

Not being as smart as most, I have had to distill the mass of data about eating behavior to terms which I can understand and remember. These principles, which are derived from years of working with behavior modification work. Try them and you will correct eating misbehavior. Not overnight, but over the long haul.

The body needs six nutrients: water, minerals, vitamins, carbohydrates, protein and fat. Claims for "special" or "magic" ingredients are good for filling the wallets of the hucksters but not for any nutritional value because of any magic. If they are absorbed and used beneficially they have the six nutrients. Nothing else!

Water

Water is the most necessary nutrient. It comprises most of our body weight. We can go for extended periods of time without the other nutrients but not so without water. It is the prime medium for transporting the things which make us tick. Muscle is more than 73 percent water.

Although water is vital to our existence, it is also the most neglected nutrient. Many times when we feel drained, energy is lacking and we feel the onset of headaches we blame any and everything when often it is the result of dehydration.

A good way to start the day is to drink a big glass of water, and repeat the drinking throughout the day. Don't wait until you get thirsty because that means you are already starting to dehydrate. Drink plenty of fluids <u>before</u> thirst. Six to eight glasses of water a day is the minimum amount recommended.

Minerals

Minerals are needed in very small amounts. It is the rare case when they are not amply provided for by eating a balanced diet. There is a definite danger in consuming too many. Don't fall for the sales pitch about taking massive doses as supplements. They can get you in trouble!

Vitamins

One of the most often asked questions is, "Should I take vitamins?" The answer is yes.

Vitamins are necessary.

Vitamins are co-enzymes. They assist enzymes in regulating the rate of metabolizing food. Contrary to popular belief, they have no food energy. There are people who take massive doses of vitamins and supplements thinking they take the place of food. They don't. Vitamins do not take the place of food. No food, no energy.

The real question is how they should be taken, and therein lies a problem.

The prevalent wisdom by the medical community and registered dieticians is that we can get all of the vitamins we need from a balanced diet. The other opinion is that the so-called normal diet should have vitamin supplements. Which position is correct?

Maybe the truth is somewhere between the two.

Apparently, mega-doses of vitamins can be harmful. There is no compelling evidence that moderate doses cause problems.

It seems that every time a definitive statement is made that we do not need vitamin supplements, a study appears, by the medical community no less, which justifies taking additional amounts of a vitamin for a specific purpose.

At various times I have convinced myself that I knew the answers. I am supposed to be reasonably well-informed on the subject, but now I am reasonably certain that I don't know the answers. I wish I could recommend a position and do it with certainty. I can't. With no claim of omnipotence, let me cautiously suggest:

1. A moderate dose vitamin supplement will probably do you no harm. It may or may not be beneficial.

2. If you purchase vitamins, buy the inexpensive kind.

3. Be smart and eat a balanced diet, with or without supplements.

4. There are supplements other than vitamins which may be of value, i.e., calcium, iron.

5. Needs vary with the individual.

6. Be cautious about "mass prescriptions."

Sorry, but that's it!

Carbohydrates

The main source of carbohydrates is from plant foods. It is our most ready and available source of energy in the form of glucose and its storage form, glycogen. Carbohydrates have fewer calories than do protein and fat. A diet high in carbohydrates is essential for adequate nutrition and fiber and is a must for sparing protein. Remember, most of the world's nutrition does not walk around, it grows!

Of course most of us are taught that we should avoid those fattening foods such as bread, potatoes, rice and the other starches. Wrong! These foods are mostly carbohydrates and carbohydrates have only 116 calories for each ounce as compared to 121 for protein and 264 for fat. Take the traditional all-American meal, meat and potatoes. Six ounces of steak could have around 500 calories. The potatoes probably have around 150 calories. From a caloric standpoint we are better off forgetting the steak and loading up on potatoes, just the opposite of what we are taught.

We need to understand two kinds of carbos, those which have - or have retained after processing - the nutrients and fiber, and those carbos which through processing have lost all or a significant portion of these nutrients. The produce counter has the first kind and the candy section has the second. Other sections of the supermarket may have varying combinations. You will most often see these two types of carbos listed as complex and simple.

Protein

Proteins are combinations of amino acids. Of the 22 amino acids, eight of them must come from dietary sources. Protein is found in both animal and plant foods. Animal protein is complete. By complete is meant that the animal source has all of the eight amino acids. Plant protein is incomplete in any one-plant source and, therefore, different plants must be eaten in combination to supply the necessary eight amino acids.

Protein's primary function is to build and repair tissue. The recommended amount for this function is .36 grams for each pound of ideal body weight.

When the body is depleted of carbohydrates, which is rare, protein is used as a fuel source resulting in tissue breakdown. Carbohydrates are also needed for fat metabolism.

Fat

Fat is the most calorie-dense food source, more than twice the calories in either carbohydrate or protein. Fat is the nutrient which has been implicated as contributing to the onset of many diseases, although in the proper amount it is necessary for the body's functions.

How Much?

How much carbohydrate, protein and fat should we consume?

No one knows and opinions vary but the most accepted recommendations are:

The percentage of daily calories should be no more than 30 percent (for weight loss, 20 percent may be more appropriate) from fat, 15 percent from protein and the remainder from carbohydrates with no more than 10 percent of these being from simple carbohydrates. In other words, as is obvious, the bulk of our diet should be from the complex carbohydrates. The diet should be low in fat, moderate in protein and high in complex carbohydrates.

Caveat: These recommendations may not suit _you_! Give them a try over a prolonged period of time. Adjust if appropriate!

Diets

The good thing about diets is that they are guaranteed. The bad thing is what they guarantee. They are guaranteed to make you fatter! Some might ask, "how can a diet of 600 calories a day make you fat?" Simple! Remember two points. When eaten, three things happen to food. First, it is used for fuel, second, it is used to build and repair tissue, and third, when the first two demands are met, the surplus intake is stored as fat. The second point to remember is that when you are on an excessively low-calorie diet a significant portion of the weight lost will be lean tissue, and the lean tissue, primarily muscles, is the calorie-burning machinery of the body.

With this information let's track a diet.

You go on a low-calorie diet. You lose weight. Forget the hype about pills, supplements and injections. They just cost you money. It's taking in fewer calories than you burn which causes weight loss, not the frills.

The weight comes off and what have you lost? You have lost fat and a good deal of the lean tissue. Now you come off of the diet. (And you <u>will</u> come off of the diet!) Will power and good intentions have nothing to do with it, it is basic biochemistry. Now that you are off of the diet you are eating as of old. The weight comes back on, it always does, but the weight you are adding is fat, not most of the lean tissue. By depleting the lean tissue you have reduced the calorie burning machinery. As a result, the fuel requirements are lowered and there is more of a surplus to be stored as fat. Now what are you? Fatter, that's what!

Worry not. Next week there will be another diet and you just know it's the one for you. You have to try it. Unfortunately, all that's for you is another cycle with the same result; you get fatter and fatter.

Each person thinks he is the one who will be the exception to the rule. It goes like this, "I know all of that. But I'll just diet down to where I want to be, level off and keep it there." Please do not deceive yourself. It's not going to happen! Of the thousands of people this author has had the privilege of working with, I have yet to see the exception.

"Breakfast Like a Queen (King), Lunch Like a Prince and Dinner Like a Pauper"

Most people have eating habits which follow an all too familiar pattern.

We arise in the a.m., hopefully, and are tired, or at least not overcome with excess energy. To get going we have to have a pick-em-up. Maybe a cup of coffee or a cola and a sweet, usually a doughnut or danish and we are on the way. We feel better. What has happened is that the caffeine and sugar cause the blood sugar (glucose) our first line of energy which is low to begin with because of having fasted during the night, to quickly exit the bloodstream and get to the central nervous system where it "picks us up." The problem is that it does not put any glucose back into the bloodstream and as soon as the initial high wears off we still have low blood sugar. A couple of hours later we need another "fix." Thus was born the Great American Coffee Break. With this latest departure of what little blood sugar is left we struggle through until lunch. For lunch we have a salad because we just know that anything else will cause a fat tumor to break out on the tummy within five minutes. Now comes the 1 p.m. to 5 p.m. blahs! These blahs may take the form of drowsiness, mood swings, irritability, etc. No problem. We go home and immediately eat the drapes, refrigerator door and dining room table. We have entered the Great American Fat Zone which is between 5 p.m. and midnight. This is the time when we consume 90 percent of the daily calories.

Remember, blood glucose levels help dictate appetite

It's the next morning. We are tired again. We should be. We have been working all night digesting food! And the cycle begins anew.

This eating pattern is disastrous. Let's reverse it.

We have been taught that breakfast is the most important meal of the day, and it is. Eat breakfast! But you say you don't care for cereals or bacon and eggs. Who said anything about breakfast food? Eat some of the same things for breakfast you normally eat for dinner. I can hear it now: "No way I can look at that stuff at that time of the morning." Of course you can't, not when you have been in the fat zone the night before. One afternoon around one o'clock run a piece of rope under you chin and tie it on top of the head so that you can not open your mouth. Leave it there until the next morning. After not being in the fat zone all night you will wake up and those chicken breasts and vegetables will look great! No kidding!

Eat a balanced breakfast. Make certain you have protein. Don't skimp on lunch. Make it balanced; carbohydrates, protein and fat. Strive to consume about 75 percent of your daily calories before 1 p.m. For the evening, eat light. After a few days you will be amazed at how much better you feel. Also, I have never known a person with a weight problem who controlled it long-term who did not stabilize his blood sugar with a good, balanced breakfast. Once again, it is not a matter of likes, dislikes or will-power, it's biochemistry.

Weight or Fat?

You don't want to lose weight! Yes, I know, all you have heard is how most of us should lose weight. Forget it, that is the last thing you need to lose. Think about it. What weight should you lose? Muscles? Not hardly. They move us and are the calorie-burning machines of the body. Not bones because when you lose the mineral density of the bone it is called osteoporosis. How about fluid, which makes up most of our weight? The fluid is absolutely essential for all of our bodily functions. Muscle is 73 percent water; without it the muscles don't work. Maybe you would like to get rid of a vital organ such as the liver or kidney; how about the brain or the heart? If you know someone who wishes to do it this way, refer them to a mental health center rather that a weight-loss clinic. So what's left? Fat. About the only calories burned by fat is the result of carrying it around. Lose the fat weight, not just weight.

Many of you don't know if you are too fat, or so you say. There are many ways to find out. Among them are skin fold calipers, underwater weighing, electrical impedance and girth circumference measures. Each method has both pluses and minuses as to accuracy. They are all estimates and often are not consistent from one measurement to another. There is one way you can check your fat which is nearly foolproof. Retire to the privacy of your bedroom and stand before a full length mirror. Disrobe and take a good long look. If you still don't know if you're too fat, jump up and down. If something wiggles and it's not supposed to, you're too fat. Enough said.

The How and The What

Distill the untold number of words down to basics and it comes to this:

How to Eat

EAT LIGHT, RIGHT and EARLY!

Light means don't overload, right means balance and early means a good breakfast and lunch!

What to Eat

This one is simple and says it all.

IF IT WALKS, BACK OFF

IF IT FLIES, USE CAUTION

IF IT SWIMS, IT'S PROBABLY OK

IF IT GROWS, EAT IT!

By backing off the walking things it tends to lower the fat intake. Flying, more accurately things which can or have flown, things are great but if overdone they can also load you up on fat.

Things which swim are usually low in fat and furnish good protein. Growing things furnish most of the world's nutrition, have the proper nutrients, are high in fiber and low in fat and therefore in calories.

This is not to say that any food group should be eliminated. Just be prudent by eating them in the recommended amounts.

Good Nutrition for Good Years

What we eat incurs consequences. Over the years the cumulative effect is evident in our quality of life. To quote L. Hofmann, "By age 65, the average American will have consumed 100,000 pounds of food, give or take a few tons. Neglect will almost certainly be reflective of his or her health by age 65, if not long before." For most of us it is <u>very</u> long before.

With advancing age the body loses active cells in each organ, although it may not be inevitable, which brings about a reduced metabolic rate. Couple this to an inactive lifestyle and the energy needs are decreased. The usual recommendation for men over 50 is 2,300 calories per day and for women 1,900 calories per day. For people over 75 the requirements are less.

Although there is a cellular loss for all of us, it is not clear how much this results in decreased energy needs for the vigorously active person. It may be minimal.

Whatever the reduced need, it is imperative that we consume foods which are dense in nutrients.

Body Sculpting and Eating Behavior

A common misconception is that building big muscles through weight training will result in significant weight and fat loss and that lean buffed look. Not so. Muscles may increase in size but they are not going to overcome excessive fat! If one wishes to achieve a sculpted appearance then the muscle-covered- fat must be reduced. This result comes from exercise (increased energy output) and appropriate eating behavior (controlled energy input).

Resistance exercise is important for long term weight control. Lean mass(muscle) burns more calories than fat. But the resistance exercise sessions do not burn as many calories as are burned during aerobic exercise. Do both!

PART 3

13
AEROBIC(ENDURANCE) EXERCISE

Twenty-one percent of that air around you is oxygen. How much and how efficiently we get those molecules of oxygen from where they are to the inside of our cells determines our energy levels, how much fat we burn and to a large degree our quality of life.

The first part of the trip is easy. The pressure difference between the atmosphere and the inside of our bronchial system transfers the oxygen to the lungs. From that point, the lungs into the cells, although pressure is still a major factor, it becomes more a matter of what we do. In other words, to a large degree we can control our oxygen supply via training.

When told that we should get as much oxygen to the cells as possible, many people assume that they should inhale long and hard. That's fine, but it will not result in much more oxygen delivery than doing nothing. And despite claims of uninformed hucksters, there is no food, diet, pill or anything else which is going to increase the oxygen delivery system in a healthy body. In fact, many complex chemical actions must take place to boost the supply of oxygen to the cell. And what can we do to influence these actions? It's called aerobic training.

The formula for aerobic training is simple: Move the major muscles for a prolonged period of time at appropriate levels of intensity!

Consider the major muscles to be those of the legs, buttocks, stomach, back and shoulders.

What is a prolonged period of time? It is not certain that there is a precise number of minutes. Remember, we are not talking about what training time is required for a specific athletic or sporting event, rather, what is adequate for improving aerobic capacity. And even that will vary depending on your level of conditioning. For the person with a high level of aerobic capacity, it may take more time at a higher intensity to show improvement than for a person with a low aerobic capacity. The standard recommendation is a minimum of 30 minutes, but in the beginning, do what you can. It may be for only a very few minutes and that's fine. When you adapt to that time of exertion you may then go to a longer time or a higher level of intensity.

And what is meant by intensity? For aerobic conditioning, use speed of movement to mean intensity. As speed of movement increases so does your number of heart beats per minute which parallels the increase in the oxygen usage. As a result, counting the number of heart beats per minute can give an indication of the intensity of an activity. (Note: An increase in heart rate during <u>anaerobic</u> exercise is not necessarily an indication of oxygen utilization.) Each of us has a maximum heart rate. It is usually recommended that we achieve between 60 and 85 percent of that maximum for an aerobic benefit. For example: if the max heart rate is 200 beats per minute, 60 percent of that is 120 heart beats per minute, 85 percent is 170 beats per minute. Another way of saying it is that you are performing at an intensity between 60 and 80 percent of your max. The lower intensities, 60-75 percent and maybe as low as 50 percent for a few, can initiate and sustain aerobic conditioning. The higher intensities may yield higher gains.

The problem is in establishing a maximum heart rate. The surest method of doing this is to undergo a physician-administered maximum stress test. It is suggested that anyone over 40, or who has a family history of cardiovascular disease, smokes or has medical problems should get a physicians clearance before undertaking an exercise program. If you do check with your physician, you may wish to request a stress test. The down side of that is the cost.

In the absence of a stress test, an accepted method is to subtract your age from 220 and then take 60 to 85 percent of that number.

Example: Age 50, 70 percent intensity

$$\begin{aligned} & 220 \\ \text{Minus} \quad & \underline{50} \\ \text{Equals} \quad & 170 \\ \text{Times} \quad & \underline{.70} \\ \text{Equals Exercise HR} \quad & 119 \end{aligned}$$

Note: Maximum heart rate goes down about one beat each year after the early 20s.

Although a good case can be made that there can be a significant error in this method, it is a good general indicator. To monitor heart rate, place the fingers lightly over either the large artery in the wrist or the large carotid artery in the neck and count for 15 seconds and multiply by four.

HEART RATE

Fifteen-Second Count Times Four

15 Sec. Count	=	1 Minute H.R.
20	=	80
21	=	84
22	=	88
23	=	92
24	=	96
25	=	100
26	=	104
27	=	108
28	=	112
29	=	116
30	=	120
31	=	124

32	=	128
33	=	132
34	=	136
35	=	140
36	=	144
37	=	148
38	=	152
39	=	156
40	=	160
41	=	164
42	=	168
43	=	172
44	=	176
45	=	180
46	=	184
47	=	188
48	=	192

Take the first heart rate after about five minutes into the exercise and again immediately upon concluding the exercise.

Another option is to monitor the rate of perceived exertion. One of the simplest ways to do this is to notice the breathing rate. When the breathing is deep and rhythmical you are in the aerobic zone. When the breathing is short and labored you are in the anaerobic zone and the intensity may be to high.

After becoming an experienced aerobic exerciser, you may not need to check your heart rate to know if you are in the proper heart rate zone. You will know by feel whether you are or not.

The exercises which utilize the large muscles range from jogging in place to running a marathon, from cycling one hundred miles to pumping a stationary bike. It may be walking, swimming, jumping rope, aerobic dancing or you-name-it. The list is endless. Which is the best? Choose the one, or several, which you will do, as long as it fits the formula. Remember, we are referring to exercises which increase energy for endurance and not necessarily those which are best for developing strength, flexibility, speed or athletic performance.

Comparing aerobic exercises, the following chart is used to illustrate that as long as the formula is adhered to, the method is secondary.

	Run	Walk	Bike	Swim
Distance	4 Mi.	4 Mi.	12 Mi.	1 Mi.
Time	40 Min.	56 Min.	48 Min.	45 Min.
Calories Used (Approx.)	400	400	400	400

The distances vary. The times are close. Intensities necessary for the times are similar. The calories expended are approximately the same. The exercises fit the formula.

Obviously, for those of us who wish to lose fat the more minutes exercised, the more calories are used.

While many exercises may fit the formula, there are differences between them which may influence your choice.

A good example is walking versus running. Walking requires that one foot always be in contact with the ground. Running means that there are phases when both feet are off the ground at the same time, which adds a vertical energy requirement to that needed for horizontal (forward) motion, and, therefore, can be slightly more energy costly than walking when done over the same period of time. That is not the same as saying the two have great differences in energy requirements over the same distance. Yes, running a mile can use more energy than walking the same distance but not a great deal more, although it may depend more on the speed chosen than the distance. For instance walking at somewhere between three-and-a-half miles an hour or faster, for most of us, is mechanically inefficient and can require a good deal more energy than an easy jog at five to six miles an hour. The result can be that a high intensity walk may be use more energy than a slow run but not a fast run. Obvious, and makes sense. So which is better for aerobic (endurance) training? It depends on the individual and the degree of intensity. For the beginner, it is probably not a good idea to start as a runner. First, condition the long-neglected muscles and joints by walking and gradually increase the intensity. When the intensity (speed) is high enough you may choose to stick with the walking as it will provide a more-than-adequate training effect, or then, if you wish, begin a running program. There is no "better" if the intensities are comparable.

Another consideration is walking or running on a treadmill. The energy cost of treadmill locomotion is considerably less than doing the same thing on a non-moving surface. On the treadmill the surface moves under you. On a non-moving surface you are expending energy pulling yourself over the distance to be covered. Also, wind resistance may come into play. Holding onto treadmill handrails will also lessen energy requirements. This is not to imply that an appropriate workout cannot be achieved on a treadmill. It simply suggests that you may have to move your legs faster, go longer, or increase the grade on a treadmill.

Biking; indoors (stationary bike) or out-of-doors? When biking outside, the major force, about 80 percent, working against you is that of air resistance. Obviously, this is not a problem inside, where the resistance is supplied by mechanical adjustment or flywheel speed. Although the physiological stresses can be equated, can the mental? Choose the one which will not bore you to wrought distraction and that you will stay with. Almost invariably people opt for the outside. An important factor in biking is saddle height. Position the saddle so that on the downstroke the leg is almost straight.

When you feel comfortable with your conditioning you may wish to try off-road biking. It's worlds of fun, is not boring and provides a great workout in a relatively short period of time.

NOTE: A lower saddle height may be desirable when biking off-road.

Many people enjoy aerobic dancing or aerobic calisthenics. Be they high or low impact, the important consideration is intensity. If the goal is fat loss and endurance development then the intensity should be moderate, and that is a pace which keeps the breathing deep and rhythmical and can be maintained for 30 minutes or more. High intensity is fine if the muscles and connective tissue are well-conditioned, but beware of the instructor who goes for the rapid pace from the beginning. As with any exercise, begin a session slowly and increase the pace gradually.

Swimming is an excellent exercise, although it may not be optimal for fat loss. Swimming is an exercise where proper mechanical form plays an important part in determining energy expenditure. If you have doubts about your swimming ability you may wish to seek the services of a competent swimming coach.

The exercises for increasing your endurance are, of course, your choice. Do the ones which you enjoy, but be certain they fit the time and intensity requirements of aerobic training.

Getting Started

Regardless of the aerobic exercise, if we start as fast as we feel like going, we are going too fast!

A natural tendency is to go too fast for the first few minutes. When we do, we pay for it later on. It takes time for the body to mobilize the various physiological functions. As they kick in, step by step, the intensity will increase keeping pace with what the body dictates. The better our aerobic conditioning, the sooner our systems allow increasing intensity. In other words, let the body warm-up and then adapt to each successive effort. You will be amazed at how much more comfortable you will feel in the latter stages of exercise.

Most problems from aerobic exercise come from trying to do too much (distance or speed) too soon. Don't!

The Timeless Exercise

To the long recognized killers such as heart disease and cancer, add AIDS and the re-emergence of tuberculosis. Another one which may affect more people than each of them is "the hurry-up sickness."

We live by the numbers and time. Be there, do this and get through. It is as if the present has no value, so hurry up and get it behind us. The only instant which matters is the next one, assuming there is one. It is a hurry-up and get-finished society.

The numbers on the clock face are supposed to tell us what to do and how well we do it. How many times a day do you check the time? Set the alarm for wake-up time, be on time for work, 30 minutes for lunch and please let knocking-off time hurry up and get here? How many times an hour do you check your watch? Attention to time results in hurrying to use it, wanting it to pass or feeling guilty about wasting it, all of which can be stressful. Too much stress results in distress, the system breaks down and hence the "hurry-up sickness."

There are 168 hours in a week and that we cannot change. What we can do is live each one as ours and enjoy them, or blast through all 168 to get them behind you. Which makes the most sense?

Time awareness is vital for science and managing the daily affairs of any society, but should it rule every aspect of our lives? Are there not times when we should "live in the moment" and not concern ourselves with how long it takes?

Because exercise should be enjoyable, ought it be governed by the clock? Maybe yes, maybe no; it depends on goals and the individual. If your personality dictates that you should measure your exercise gains by how long it takes to complete a given activity, then use the clock. If this is not your priority, then don't use it.

Almost every aerobic exercise program includes a time goal. This is fine, it can motivate and is a way of keeping score. It also can create a sense of failure when time limits are not met and lead to excessive pressure to "do well."

Exercise can be effective, and often more enjoyable, when it is done in accordance with the body's clock rather than a manufactured one.

Let us consider an example of an aerobic exercise done without a clock and, therefore, in accord with the way our bodies work physiologically.

Distance running. If we wish to better adhere to the way our bodies work we would begin the distance with a comfortable walk followed by a fast walk. Then would come a slow jogging shuffle, slowly picking up the tempo until achieving the fastest comfortable pace which allows us to finish the distance. And when should we transition from one speed to the next fastest speed? When the body is ready! As the muscles become warm and the oxygen transport system is activated, intensity of activity increases. Each level of intensity becomes easier.

Aerobic exercise can be done, obviously, with or without a watch. For many people it is more enjoyable when done without reference to the time it takes. If the goal is to train for competition, then watching the clock is the way to go. A variation of these approaches is to train a set distance without a time goal and then periodically check your time, maybe once a month.

Alternatives are:

    1. Go without a distance or time goal

    2. Go a measured distance without a time goal

3. Set a time goal not related to distance

4. Go for a set distance with a time goal

Approximately 100 calories are burned for each mile walked or run. Figure to use about 100 calories each 12 minutes biked at 4:30 per mile. Swimming 12 minutes at a 1:20 pace for each 50 yards (One pool lap) requires about 100 calories.

Increases in aerobic capacity occur slowly. The most rapid improvements happen in the beginning of training. Afterwards, the gains come much slower. Be patient.

The most evident result of endurance training is the increase in energy levels.

14
AEROBIC HOW-TO

<u>READ CAREFULLY BECAUSE YOU ARE GOING TO BE SURPRISED!</u>

Exercise charts which say do this exercise for this heart rate this many times a week is like counting calories; it is a pain in the "uh huh" and no one is going to do either on a daily basis for a prolonged period of time. Why should we? Why do something which is no fun - maybe boring - and additionally get over-anxious about numbers? Instead, let's try it the natural way; the way people did it before we got so hung up on thinking we have to be miserable in order to be worthy and fit.

NOTE: This is not to say that if you enjoy doing it by the numbers you should not. Just the contrary, but be aware of the option.

THINK F.I.T.T.

Frequency: * Standard Recommendation: no fewer than three days each week.

* Best Interpretation: Start with a frequency you can live with and work up to the standard. It doesn't have to be the same number of times each and every week.

* Long-Term Functional Recommendation: As often as you want to. If it turns out that the frequency is not often enough or is too often - you'll know. Your body will tell you.

Intensity:
* Standard Recommendation: Fast enough to get the heart rate up to between 65% and 85 % of your maximum heart rate.

*Best Interpretation: Make the breathing deep and rythmical. If the breathing gets harsh and labored, slow down.

* Long-Term Functional Recommendation: When the intensity gets too high (too strenuous to be enjoyable), back off. When you have recovered start increasing it to the point where you can sustain it for as long as you wish.

Time:
* Standard Recommendation: At least 20 to 30 minutes.

* Best Interpretation: Can be in small chunks. You may wish to go for two or three minutes, recover and do another two or three. As things get better you can put the small chunks together or raise the short time intensity.

* Long-Term Functional Recommendation: Listen to your body. Go for whatever time you can. When miserable, bored or too tired - stop.

Type:
* Standard Recommendation: Do aerobic exercises. Huh? What are they?

* Best Interpretation: Intensity determines whether a movement is aerobic or anaerobic, not the exercise!

*Long-Term Functional Recommendation: Do one or a combination of exercises that you enjoy. No law says you have to pick just one exercise. If you wish, do different ones on different days or even on the same day.

NOTE: Some of the more familiar ones which can be done at the appropriate intensity are:

    Walking

    Running

    Biking

    Swimming

Remember the Rule?

MOVE THE MAJOR MUSCLES RHYTHMICALLY FOR A PROLONGED PERIOD OF TIME AT THE APPROPRIATE INTENSITY.

If you wish to utilize a more quantified schedule of aerobic training I suggest Dr. Ken Cooper's book "AEROBICS."

Or, contact me Don McDaniel, 1-850-478-0475

E-mail: mcd@pcola.gulf.net

15

POWER AND ENDURANCE

After appropriate conditioning with resistance training, usually several weeks, add the endurance training of your choice.

Gradually improve to the point where you are doing resistance training at least three days each week along with three days of endurance training.

When the six workouts should be scheduled is a matter of preference, condition and the time needed for recovery. Any number of combinations may be appropriate.

Allow at least one day between resistance training sessions and train for endurance no more than two consecutive days, once again, dependent upon workout intensity.

If the intensity is light to moderate, both resistance and endurance training can be done on the same days.

Because each of us responds to exertion in different ways and recovery times vary, it takes a time of trial and error before we know which schedule fits our needs. Do not hesitate to change the schedule!

"REST IS A WEAPON"

Sun Tzu (circa A.D. 700)

Exercise is a stimulate. For stimulation to be effective, resulting in training progress, there must be adaptation to the stimulus. Adaptation requires time. The rest between exercise sessions is the time when progress occurs.

Often we become enamored with the idea that the more we do the better we become. More is not always better. Doing too much can become counter-productive. Take time to adapt. Take time to recover!

If you feel fatigued, you are not ready for another exercise session. Listen to your body.

Most of the time exercise into <u>exhilaration</u>, not exhaustion!

FOR ALL OF US
LIVING AT ANY AGE

* Love each other
* Laugh
* Don't take ourselves too seriously
* Stay loose
* Increase muscle power
* Train to endure
* Eat sensibly
* Strive to be capable of doing whatever you need or

Thanks for sharing your time.

Sincerely,

Don McDaniel

NOTES

NOTES

Printed in the United States
1534000001B/29-52